SARS

IN CONTEXT

MEMORY, HISTORY, POLICY

McGill-Queen's/Associated Medical Services Studies in the History of Medicine, Health, and Society

Series Editors: S.O. Freedman and J.T.H. Connor

Volumes in this series have financial support from Associated Medical Services, Inc. (AMS). Associated Medical Services Inc. was established in 1936 by Dr Jason Hannah as a pioneer prepaid not-for-profit health care organization in Ontario. With the advent of medicare, AMS became a charitable organization supporting innovations in academic medicine and health services, specifically the history of medicine and health care, as well as innovations in health professional education and bioethics.

SARS

IN CONTEXT

MEMORY, HISTORY, POLICY

EDITED BY

JACALYN DUFFIN AND
ARTHUR SWEETMAN

The School of Policy Studies, Queen's University
McGill-Queen's University Press
Montreal and Kingston • London • Ithaca

© McGill-Queen's University Press 2006

ISBN-13: 978-0-7735-3194-9   ISBN-10: 0-7735-3194-7 (paper)
ISBN-13: 978-0-7735-3193-2   ISBN-10: 0-7735-3193-9 (cloth)

Legal deposit fourth quarter 2006
Bibliothèque nationale du Québec

Printed in Canada on acid-free paper.

McGill-Queen's University Press acknowledges the support of the Canada Council for the Arts for our publishing program. We also acknowledge the financial support of the Government of Canada through the Book Publishing Industry Development Program (BPIDP) for our publishing activities.

Library and Archives Canada Cataloguing in Publication

     SARS in context : memory, history, policy / edited by Jacalyn Duffin and Arthur Sweetman.

(McGill-Queen's/Associated Medical Services studies in the history of medicine,
     health, and society ; 27)
Includes bibliographical references and index.
ISBN-13: 978-0-7735-3193-2 (bound)
ISBN-13: 978-0-7735-3194-9 (pbk.)
ISBN-10: 0-7735-3193-9 (bound)
ISBN-10: 0-7735-3194-7 (pbk.)

     1. SARS (Disease)—Ontario—Epidemiology—History—21st century.
2. Communicable diseases—Ontario—History. I. Duffin, Jacalyn
II. Sweetman, Arthur III. Queen's University (Kingston, Ont.). School of
Policy Studies IV. Series.

RA644.S17.S276 2006   614.5'92   C2006-902995-4

To the memory of those who died of SARS

CONTENTS

TABLES AND FIGURES

ACKNOWLEDGEMENTS

We are grateful for the support of Dean David M.C. Walker, the Hannah Chair of the History of Medicine, and the Stauffer-Dunning Chair at Queen's University at Kingston, and for the help of Marilyn Banting, Mark Howes, Valerie Jarus, Joshua Lipton-Duffin, and Cherrilyn Yalin.

An earlier version of the chapter, "Governance in Pandemics: Defining the Federal Government's Role in Public Health Emergencies," by Kumanan Wilson and Harvey Lazar previously appeared as "Planning for the Next Pandemic Threat: Defining the Federal Role in Public Health Emergencies," in *Policy Matters* (Vol. 6, no. 5, 2005), published by the Institute for Research on Public Policy (IRPP). We thank IRPP for permission to include the current version in book form here.

ABOUT THE COVER

Protection from infection?

An eighteenth-century plague doctor wears gown, mask, and gloves to prevent contagion and reduce the stench of infected or dead bodies. The stick provides distance from patients as he works. From Jean-Jacques Manget, *Traité de la peste* (Geneva, 1721). The World Health Organization, based in Geneva, has digitized this work at http://whqlibdoc.who.int/rare-books/a56993.pdf.

"SARS Ballet," 27 April 2003, award-winning photograph by Vincent Yu (b. 1964) of *Associated Press*. The Hong Kong children perform their dance poignantly masked for protection against the new pathogen that eventually affected over 1,700 people in their city, killing 299.

For more on barriers for plague and for SARS, see inside this book, pages 43-68.

1

INTRODUCTION: LESSONS AND DISAPPOINTMENTS

Jacalyn Duffin

S evere Acute Respiratory Syndrome (SARS) began in China in November 2002 and rapidly swept the globe to appear on five continents. From February to July 2003, it affected over 8,000 people worldwide, leaving 774 dead (including 349 in China, 299 in Hong Kong, 44 in Canada, 37 in Taiwan, and 33 in Singapore).[1] This highly contagious lung infection had a predilection for health-care workers and its victims included doctors, nurses, and their family members. The causative agent was quickly identified through international collaboration as a new strain of coronavirus, SARS CoV; it was sequenced by the Michael Smith Genome Sciences Centre in British Columbia helped by the BC Centre for Disease Control and Winnipeg's National Microbiology Laboratory.[2] Tracked by extraordinary media coverage, control of the outbreak of this novel pathogen was achieved through ancient methods: strict isolation of sufferers and quarantine of their contacts. SARS taxed the chronically underfunded public health services of several countries and in its wake left many other sequelae: medical, social, political, economic, and legislative.

The outbreak made heavy demands on public health workers and infectious disease specialists. In Canada, cases appeared in Vancouver and Toronto. Few people outside the country realize that hospitals across the entire province of Ontario were quarantined during the acute phase. Restrictions on hospital activities and visitors remained in place for weeks, resulting in emotional turmoil. New rituals of hand-washing and temperature monitoring were implemented. In addition to its direct costs, SARS also resulted in massive economic disruption to Canada's largest city, a situation aggravated by the World Health Organization (WHO) travel advisories. Travellers from Asia and people of Asian origin experienced outright discrimination. Even as the consumption of face masks escalated, SARS served to unmask flaws in the existing safety net for infection control; and it highlighted our continued vulnerability to natural pathogens. The disease occurred only in two Canadian cities, but its legislative impact is felt on a national scale. Looking back, many experts believe that we escaped a devastating pandemic more by good luck than by good management.

This volume is not a history of SARS. The authors recount some events of the outbreak as needed for their observations; however, anyone looking for a fuller chronology is encouraged to consult the three reports on the management and implications of SARS in Canada,[3] or summaries in the medical literature,[4] or the Web sites sponsored by the WHO[5] and the Canadian Broadcasting Corporation (CBC).[6] The latter site offers links to online versions of the major reports. A journalistic history by Thomas Abraham gives a good account of events outside Canada.[7]

Instead, this volume consists of individual reflections on SARS from scientific, historical, economic, and policy perspectives. Most of the chapters were first read at a symposium held at Queen's University in February 2004 — a symposium that originated in the encounters of medical historians with journalists reporting on SARS.

ARE NEW DISEASES GOOD FOR OLD HISTORIANS?

In the life of a medical historian, years — even decades — can roll by without a single call from a journalist. Come a new disease, however, especially a contagious one, and medical historians are bombarded with appeals from the media seeking "lessons from the past." Historical insight was invoked at the advent of Legionnaires' disease, toxic shock syndrome, AIDS, BSE, the Ebola threats, West Nile, and the mercifully rare recrudescence of older scourges such as influenza, polio, cholera, and plague. It happened again with SARS in early 2003.

For historians of medicine, SARS brought interviews with large dailies and air-time on national television and radio. The public exposure may have been "good" for the visibility of medical history, but sometimes, the historians were forced into the uncomfortable, if not impossible position of trying to predict the future. Reporters often seemed disappointed by our responses; some lessons from the past are unwelcome. By late spring 2003, delegates at the annual medical history meetings in both Canada and the United States acknowledged the special attention that SARS had brought their way with self-deprecating amusement and grim irony: "Here we go again." It is painful to be a source of repeated disappointment. When the health danger waned with the departure of SARS, the temporary popularity of the historians waned too.

THOSE DISAPPOINTING LESSONS FROM THE PAST

In most cases, the journalist who contacts a historian is fired up with the originality of his or her idea. Quickly, they discover that three media people have already called that day. This minor chagrin is only the first disappointment of many.

The next disappointment stems from the shortest and best answer to the inevitable question: "Can lessons from the past prevent future epidemics?" No. Nature will constantly find new ways to surprise and challenge us. "But," the journalist persists, "aren't we safer now with all our technology than we were in the past?" The answer again is "No, not really, although we are much better informed." On these matters, the medical scientists who contributed to this volume agree with the historians.

Then there are sobering lessons about loss. We mourn the health-care professionals who died in the SARS epidemic with deep respect. History teaches us that, when confronted with an unknown, new disease, good care-giving could mean that, on occasion, doctors and nurses will sicken, even die, along with their patients. This discouraging lesson pales in contrast to another: medical cowardice will arise. For every valiant doctor who died from the disease being fought, another ran away. Flight from apparent contagion — a sane reflex for self-preservation — is prehistoric in origin. But it has always been limited in scope: fraught with danger in wartime, it is available only to the privileged during peace. Physicians ought not to shun the needy, but we know that great doctors, including both Galen and Thomas Sydenham, are said to have fled epidemics when they realized that medicine was of no avail.[8] With SARS and also with AIDS, doctors try to avoid risk by resorting to controversial mechanisms: for example, we disapprove of (but tolerate) refusal to treat HIV-infected patients for elective procedures. In a crisis, norms of "correct" behaviour are tossed aside.

To illustrate these points, historians often refer to the account of the "Plague of Athens," written by the Greek historian, Thucydides, in the fifth century BC. So reliably is this text trotted out at the advent of a new disease (or a new outbreak of an old disease), just as I am doing now, that a "plague year" can be identified by an increase in the "Thucydides Index," or the number of references to Thucydides in the *Science Citation Index.*[9] Long a temptation for retrospective diagnosticians, the Plague of Athens has been attributed to the organisms that cause typhus, smallpox, anthrax, toxic shock, and AIDS. Given the millennia that have passed since it appeared and the mutability of biological forms, and lacking any human remains or any written accounts (other than that of Thucydides), the exact "diagnosis" of the Athenian plague is probably unknowable. A more important lesson from this ancient text is in its context of circumstances and reactions. War and deprivation fostered the epidemic. Surprise, suspicion, and xenophobia heralded its arrival. Feebly enforced rules for hygiene and travel emerged in its midst. And legislative insubordination, chaos, and anger swirled in its wake. Brave caregivers died; wiser ones fled.

Sound familiar? Fill in the blank with respect to diagnosis and the perennial scenario has been played over and over again through time and place, another of history's great disappointments. We seem to be no smarter nor any kinder than our distant predecessors.

QUARANTINE: THE TYRANNY OF NEGATIVE EVIDENCE

The most poignant phone call that I received during the SARS outbreak came from a public health officer, exhausted from his front-line labours. He had the difficult task of justifying the quarantine of numerous, seemingly healthy people, to politicians, journalists, and citizens. The critics doubted its need and its value, and they railed against its human and monetary costs. "Some concrete examples might help," he said wearily. "Did quarantine ever work?"

The annoying but true answer to that question is "sometimes." The word "quarantine" is derived from "quarante" (forty), the number of days in Lent, which symbolically commemorates Christ's self-imposed sojourn in the wilderness. Isolation of the sick may be an ancient practice, but segregation of healthy travellers was first encoded in the fourteenth century, when it was invoked to "control" plague in the port cities of Ragusa (now Dubrovnik) and Venice. This mechanism was predicated on the notion of contact. With no conceptual role for germs, fleas, or rats at that time, it is easy to see how breaches in the system occurred and the disease sometimes spread.

In nineteenth-century North America, quarantine of immigrants against typhus and cholera entailed confining healthy travellers together with the sick in unsanitary quarters, often on islands. The death toll included thousands who might never have fallen ill had the sick people been housed separately. And the pestilence crept into towns anyway. Again, it is disturbing to imagine that these measures were not only ineffective, perhaps they were worse than doing nothing. In a sense, those quarantines may have "worked" to increase mortality.

We believe that we have more ethical, and hopefully safer, ways of implementing quarantine, and sometimes it is accepted without question. For example, many people remained healthy in the pre-vaccine outbreaks of mumps and polio during the 1930s, 1940s, and early 1950s. Which of the lucky "survivors" who did not fall ill would dare to argue that quarantine played no role in sparing them from death or the ravages of disability owing to those great diseases? Similarly, the hardy, smaller-scale measures for treating (as well as segregating) those exposed to meningitis provoke little outcry and result in compliance.

But when quarantine is invoked on a large, impersonal scale, its economic consequences generate self-righteous anger and unfair exceptions. Powerful élites perceive threats to their wealth and aspirations; they pretend that quarantine is doubly useless — in theory, because the "real" causes are unknown, and in practice, because the masses cannot be trusted to follow recommendations. We heard these arguments during the SARS crisis.

To my friend in public health, I replied that we cannot put names and faces to those people who remained healthy because of past quarantines. Nor, alas, can we count them. Our science is enslaved to numbers and statistical modes of communicating "facts." In the absence of names, faces, and bodies, there are no numbers. This is the tyranny of negative evidence. Costly quarantine invites questions about the dollar value of human lives, questions that cannot be answered without the kind of information that our science recognizes as good evidence. Consequently, those, who are unwilling to make expensive sacrifices for literally countless, unknown others, will claim that quarantine does not work, as they have always done.

Yet when contagion is obvious, cause unknown, and vaccine or treatment lacking, venerable quarantine makes good sense. To some ears, this lesson too was unwelcome. For the scientific contributors to this volume it is a fact.

WHO IS THE WHO?

In the midst of the outbreak, I was both horrified and intrigued that my media contacts, prompted by the then mayor of Toronto, Mel Lastman, began to ask, "Isn't it time to get rid of the WHO? Hasn't it been outmoded by our new technologies and pharmaceuticals?" Here again, the answer was an obvious "No!" Vexed with that reply, the reporters would counter with another question: "But what good is the WHO when it is obviously doing serious [economic] harm?" Once again, stories from the past helped to explain.

Take the pre-WHO example of influenza in 1918, often unfairly called the "Spanish flu." Many theories account for its appearance. Recent scholarship, using a wide array of methods, suggests that influenza may have originated as early as 1916 in France, or in China, or even on hog farms in the American mid-west and circled the globe once, possibly twice, before Spain became the first country to declare the epidemic. A non-combatant, Spain was not under security restrictions on information imposed by wartime hostilities.[10] Might we imagine that some lives could have been spared from influenza had the WHO been in existence in 1918?

From a history perspective, the WHO was founded only a short time ago. Still, it was instrumental in the global eradication of smallpox; it is on a fast track for eliminating polio. True, some of its projects resulted in defeat, even harm, witness its DDT-driven attempt to eradicate malaria. The WHO strives to collect and disseminate data with what is hoped to be impartiality. To those objecting to the Toronto travel advisory, I replied (ironically, from Toronto) that the WHO was simply doing its job. Confronted with a serious outbreak of a dangerous new disease, the WHO could tell you which places to avoid if you did not want to die of SARS.

As James Young's statistics later showed, the WHO may have closed the barn door too tightly and too late. His colleague, Dick Zoutman, wonders about how well-intentioned transparency, fostered by the desire to share information, contributed to that decision. In the heat of the moment and faced with the threat of global disease, on which side of caution should authorities err?

But the WHO knows that we will all die of something. It tracks many other diseases too. The journalists could visit the WHO Web site to learn where *not* to go to avoid malaria, dengue, Ebola, diarrhea, influenza, cholera, and AIDS; some of those diseases kill millions every year. Because we understand how to manage and treat those outbreaks, should we not campaign to lift travel advisories to those places too? And if we are unwilling to suppress this information as it pertains to "them" in Africa or Asia, why should it be suppressed for "us" in the First World?

Imperfect though it may be, the WHO is one of those newer responses to the challenges of global health. It tries to serve as a neutral clearing house for information, which itself is a valuable weapon in the control of epidemics. This admittedly conservative response also disappointed the reporters.

PATHOCENOSIS: QUESTIONS THAT ARE NOT ASKED

The causative agent of the SARS epidemic was isolated and characterized quickly as a new type of coronavirus. These RNA-viruses are named for the "crown-like" appearance of the outer envelope of the virus as seen under an electron microscope. First derived from chickens in the 1930s, they were previously thought to produce colds and mild respiratory infections in humans.[11] The rapidity of this scientific achievement for SARS was reminiscent of efforts to identify the cause of Legionnaire's disease back in the 1970s, and it stood in contrast to the slowness of finding the AIDS pathogen in the early 1980s. Historians accept that socio-cultural differences between the AIDS population and those afflicted with other more "respectable" diseases contributed to a relative delay in the race to identify HIV; the barriers were technical, conceptual, ethical, and political. With SARS, we were lucky. But the causes of a disease do not end with isolating the virus.

The cause of any disease is more than the necessary biological agent, the presence of which may not be sufficient for an outbreak. Causes also include social factors, such as war and poverty, and natural disasters, such as earthquakes and flooding, population age, other illnesses, travel, and lifestyle, including sexual, dietary, and cultural practices. Controlling these factors has sometimes been enough to stop an epidemic.

For example, smallpox control through vaccinia (cowpox) was discovered in the late eighteenth century by Edward Jenner, long before either virus (variola or vaccinia) had been isolated. Similarly in the 1850s, decades before germ theory, John Snow stopped a cholera outbreak in London by removing the handle of a water pump. For Snow, the cause had been water from that particular pump. In the case of tuberculosis, the decline in mortality from 1800 forward is said to have owed more to rising individual wealth and public health measures than it did to the discovery of the bacillus, the vaccines, and the drugs.

One cause of new diseases is a window of opportunity in the ecology of existing diseases. Mirko Drazen Grmek coined the word *pathocenosis* to describe the constellation of diseases affecting a certain place, at a certain time.[12] Sometimes, we can almost predict what diseases should be where and when; their absence becomes an intriguing puzzle. If one disease drops out of the scenario, it leaves a pathocenotic "hole," into which another, new (or seemingly new) pathogen can move. These holes are excavated by natural decline in virulence, or by shifts in social conditions; more disturbing is the possibility that they can also be carved out by medical science.

Now what of SARS and pathocenosis? For many years, we have been immunizing against childhood diseases and influenza. And for decades, we have worried about resistant organisms spawned by the overuse of antibiotics. Have we created a pathocenotic hole with our vaccines and our drugs? Should we have been surprised when a dangerous new respiratory infection came along? Could SARS be an inevitable product of our very science and privilege?

Reporters did not ask this question. Sometimes, however, I asked it of them, exasperated by the silver-lining, wishful thinking that pervaded their well-meaning efforts to contrast a glorious, safe present with a deprived and dirty past. History cannot reveal to what extent SARS may have been caused by modern science and technology; however, history reminds us to consider that possibility. Just one more discouraging lesson from the past.

ABOUT THIS VOLUME

In response to our common experiences, we gathered at Queen's University for a symposium on 10 and 11 February 2004, not yet a year after SARS first came to Toronto. The audience consisted of one-hundred first-year medical students, joined by 50 others from the university and the general public. Among the speakers were three physicians who had been deeply involved with the acute phase of the Toronto outbreak and were still engaged with its aftermath. Nine historians spoke about SARS in light of their expertise in disease history, and they also spoke about their ongoing research on disease history in light of SARS.[13] Policy views were expressed by health economist, Arthur Sweetman. During the symposium, students placed suggestions for good examination questions in a box; in April, they answered a question selected from their own contributions.[14] The discussion generated by each paper had an impact on the written versions that appear here.

This volume is divided into three sections. Part One, on Memory, contains the recollections of two physicians involved in managing the outbreak. James Young, former coroner of Ontario who was commissioner of safety, emphasizes that the greatest challenge as SARS emerged was recognizing it as a completely new disease and distinguishing it from all similar diseases in the community.[15] Dick Zoutman writes about how he came to chair a scientific committee tasked with advising hospitals and citizens. They describe the lived experience of the outbreak, the uncertainty, the fear, the stress, and the importance of sticking to the "rules" — even when they must be applied to the people who created them.

Both physicians are candid about the frustrations of working within the competing confines of several, well-intentioned provincial, national, and global institutions. They are deeply aware that the rules — those measures used to contain the outbreak — were traditional and had been laid down decades earlier. They also remind us that modern technology cannot prevent nature from surprising us with new and lethal challenges.

Part Two, on History, contains the reflections of five established historians of medicine, each of whom has published on epidemic diseases. They were encouraged to describe how history led them to regard the SARS outbreak, and how SARS may have altered their perspectives on the past.

Historian of plagues Ann Carmichael concentrates on the parallels and differences between SARS of 2003 and the plague epidemics of the fourteenth century. On the one hand, tracking SARS highlights the things we cannot know about plague: the absence of sources, skewed evidence in scarce records; and the risks of making assumptions about a new disease based on old ones. She opens with a detailed description of the outbreak in China and then explores two facets shared by SARS and plague: the dilemma of recognizing when a new disease has arisen (something that had also preoccupied James Young);

and the striking congruities in response modalities, notably quarantine, ritual-ized hand-washing, and the barrier technologies of gowns, gloves, and masks.

Philosopher and historian K. Codell Carter reminds us of the impor-tance of the epistemic setting that embraces any new disease as it enters the world stage. The causal context for new diseases changed markedly between 1835 and 1880. The first observers of SARS were committed to the idea of a single pathogen as a cause for new infectious diseases. But the first observers of medieval plague, early modern syphilis, and early nineteenth-century chol-era or typhus did not commit to a single universal cause, because the concept was unavailable. The "correct" search for apparent causes in those remote epi-demics was far wider, more eclectic, and more personalized. When confronted with SARS, as Dick Zoutman recalls, officials immediately began to filter in-formation through the model of a single universal cause: they assumed the cause of SARS would prove to be a virus. Recognizing the decided advantages of this perspective, especially in the SARS outbreak, Carter speculates on its limitations and possible shortcomings. Indeed, the pathogen is necessary for an outbreak, but is it always sufficient? And is it possible that all-important sufficient causes may lie outside the box, in the realm of politics, society, and culture?

Historian of public health, Heather MacDougall compares the Toronto SARS outbreak to policy aspects of the Canadian experience with other dis-eases in the past, in particular cholera, typhus, smallpox, and influenza. Each outbreak left its own unique mark on public attitudes and on the institutional structures for dealing with disease. Early in the nineteenth century, the cholera and typhus epidemics provided object lessons in the development of public policy. By the late nineteenth century, optimism that science would eventually identify the causes of all infectious diseases lent great authority to experts whose work intersected with the domain of governmental responsibility. The powerful demands of safety for the masses clashed with the ideal of preserv-ing individual lifestyle freedoms. But from cholera to polio, MacDougall shows how Toronto Public Health dealt with opposition, tried to interact with senior levels of government, took a leadership role, and generally worked with the support and approval of the public. Responses to epidemics produce new and lasting structures that linger, for better or for worse, to confront the next crisis. At the advent of SARS, Toronto had not confronted epidemic disease for half a century, and the structures had been allowed to languish. Inevitably, however, any new crisis will be something that was unimagined by previous experience, even when institutions are carefully maintained. Ironically then, the successes of earlier campaigns resulted in changes that contributed to lack of preparedness for SARS.

Historian of health policy, Georgina Feldberg opens her chapter with questions about the ways in which newspapers used the history of infections during the SARS outbreak. Tuberculosis was conspicuously absent from the media accounts. On the surface, this silence might be explained by the evident lack of similarity between the transient, acute SARS outbreak and the ancient, chronic scourge of tuberculosis. Yet, her comparison of the human reactions to these problems resulted in some surprising parallels. In both situations, the media turned to history, as if a crisis affords a natural opportunity to look back. Like Carter, Feldberg emphasizes the lasting impact of germ theory on the intellectual milieu that greeted SARS; like MacDougall, she describes the problems that arise when disease containment infringed on lifestyle. And she reminds us, once again, that causes include much more than the necessary "germ": the 1990s' rise in tuberculosis incidence in New York City was a product of the germ, yes, but also of poverty, homelessness, and another infectious agent: HIV.

Historian Jay Cassel, in reflecting on the history of sexually transmitted diseases and AIDS, also notices how the impulse to protect society will conflict with individual freedoms, even when efforts are made to avoid stereotyping. While behaviour may constitute a significant "cause" of disease — and its alteration suggests a reasonable mechanism for control — behaviour modification is difficult to sell and even more difficult to sustain. Similarly with SARS, as Young and Zoutman indicate, a second wave was tracked to the utter fatigue of hospital personnel with the rigours of stringent regulations over a relatively short, intense period of time. Little wonder, then, that sexually transmitted diseases persist: the behaviours are intimate, the controls intrusive, and the need permanent.

Part Three, on Policy, addresses policy concerns regarding epidemics from a very broad perspective. It starts with an overview of issues related to economic epidemiology and infectious diseases by Arthur Sweetman. One of the major contributions of economic epidemiology is to emphasize the importance of, and begin to formally model, behavioural responses to the threat of infection. The role of the public demand for prevention is introduced by focusing on the concept of "prevalence-elasticity": in a crisis, many individuals take extraordinary measures to protect themselves and their families. If public policy provides good information on prevalence and on how to avoid infection, this desire to self-protect can be a powerful tool for prevention. This tendency was seen in the SARS crisis when people began to wear masks in public spaces. However, the converse is also the case: when an infection has a low prevalence, few are willing to undertake even small measures, such as vaccination; in that setting, eradication or prevention will be more difficult. Some perhaps unexpected implications also flow from this model's view of the world; for example, subjective self-assessments of the probability of already being infected can have substantial impacts on behaviour and disease transmission. The example of the Plague of Athens, cited above, illustrates this point.

A second topic addressed by Sweetman is the cost of infections, especially the costs to society at large, and the implications of increasing globalization for these costs.

Finally, Sweetman considers both the trade-offs between public health, individual health, and non-health priorities in policy-making and the heterogeneity of tastes regarding the desirability of alternative outcomes. The example of highway speed limits is used to illustrate the health risks that society is willing to bear: like many epidemic and public health-related policies, highway speed limits impose a single rule for the entire population (e.g., 100, or in some provinces 120, km/hr). Almost ubiquitously, whatever rule is adopted will be found both too unsafe *and* too needlessly protective. In the case of a national health-care system, this heterogeneity of individual preferences poses special challenges for policy-making.

In the next contribution, intergovernmental relations expert Harvey Lazar and physician Kumanan Wilson use the SARS experience to propose modifications of Canada's federal legislation in order to facilitate the governance and management of future public health emergencies. They point to the increasing importance of globalization and the benefits of international coordination in motivating their proposal. They criticize the disproportionate focus of the federal government's post-SARS reforms of public health governance on developing "collaborative" intergovernmental relationships. While they support the notion of collaboration, they also see a need for federal leadership in a national emergency when the intergovernmental mechanisms may prove to be either too sluggish or relatively ineffective. In particular, they highlight the insufficiencies of the existing federal *Emergencies Act*, especially as it would apply to the early stages of an outbreak. Instead, they propose alternative, re-designed legislation that will act to (i) allow the federal government to intervene at an early stage when the ability to control the outbreak is greatest; (ii) ensure that the federal government has full information on the outbreak for communication with all provinces/territories; and (iii) enable Canada to meet its reporting obligations as outlined in the new International Health Regulations of the WHO. Some aspects of the new legislation would, however, serve only as a contingency, since, ideally, existing collaborative relationships should work effectively in a time of crisis. Moreover, the threat of contingency action may facilitate collaborative relationships. The authors also suggest a federally sponsored cost-sharing schedule that would serve to mitigate disease transmission, facilitate information flows, and increase preventative preparation, because the federal government can alleviate under-investment by provinces that do not recognize the costs that their (in)actions impose on other jurisdictions.

In the last chapter, economists Steven James and Timothy Sargent address the economic impact of historical influenza pandemics and SARS. Fully recognizing the wrenching human and social costs of a pandemic, they focus on the aggregate economic impacts. Relatively few economic studies have compared estimates made near the time of a crisis to actual historical outcomes when they eventually become available. In contrast to most in-crisis estimates, national economic and related data reveal only modest and short-term effects on aggregate macroeconomic indicators, such as industrial production, business activity, mass transit use, import and export levels, and retail sales.

James and Sargent argue that advanced economies are fairly resilient to natural shocks. The dire forecasts during and after SARS were widely endorsed by the outpouring of support for Toronto on 30 July 2003: nearly half a million people spent 15 hours in blistering heat at the 11-act outdoor concert featuring the Rolling Stones. But the predictions of large aggregate economic impacts tended not to allow for behavioural responses by firms and workers. However, without denying the enormous financial and human costs borne by some individuals, it appears that people and firms adapted to control the size of the aggregate economic impacts. Moreover, the short duration of many historical influenza pandemics and SARS also limited their macroeconomic impacts. Their analysis shows that some narrowly defined sectors may be clearly affected for a time by a pandemic, but most are not. For one surprising example from the SARS outbreak, even restaurant receipts in Ontario, relative to the rest of Canada, were not appreciably affected. Overall, in a calm after-the-fact analysis, the macroeconomic impacts of the pandemics studied appear not to be as large as was popularly anticipated, especially when the predictions were made during, or shortly after the crisis itself. A lesson that does not disappoint.

Diseases have personalities. Sometimes the personality is characterized by its principal symptoms: in that sense, SARS most resembles influenza, as an airborne, respiratory infection. Sometimes a disease takes on the "traits" of presumed sufferers who become vulnerable to stigmatization. Sometimes the personality derives from the time and place in which the disease appeared — intellectually, politically, and environmentally. These clinical and cultural differences matter, and they will dictate the shape of responses constructed in the aftermath. Thus, the identity of any new disease is shaped by the diseases that precede it, and also by the imaginations of those who are forced to confront it and prepare for the future.

While diseases may differ one from another, these essays also show that human reactions to new diseases are relentlessly constant. Furthermore, ancient measures of control remain effective even as they continue to evoke frustrating conflict between individuals and collectives, and between economic realities and moral or emotional worth. Finally, not all the lessons are disappointing: with other diseases of the past, SARS instructs us in the timeless virtues of caring, courage, inventiveness, honesty, and patience.

NOTES

[1]World Health Organization (WHO), "Communicable Disease Surveillance and Response, SARS" (Geneva: WHO, 21 April 2004). At www.who.int/csr/sars/country/table2004_04_21/en/.

[2]The announcement came on 12 April 2003. See Marco A. Marra, Steven J. Jones, Caroline R. Astell et al., "The Genome Sequence of the SARS-associated Coronavirus," Science 300, no. 5624 (2003):1399-404. See also the BC Centre for Disease Control at www.bccdc.org.

[3]C. David Naylor, Learning from SARS: Renewal of Public Health in Canada. Report of the National Advisory Committee on SARS and Public Health (Ottawa: Public Health Agency of Canada, 2003). At www.phac-aspc.gc.ca/publicat/sars-sras/naylor/.

Ontario Expert Panel on SARS and Infectious Disease Control (Dr. David Walker, chair), For the Public's Health: A Plan of Action. Final Report (Toronto: Ontario Ministry of Health and Long Term Care, April 2004).

Independent SARS Commission (Mr. Justice Archie Campbell, chair), *SARS and Public Health in Ontario,* Interim Report (Toronto: The Commission, April 2004). Independent SARS Commission, *SARS and Public Health Legislation* (Toronto: The Commission, April 2005).

[4]D.M. Skowronski, C. Astell, R.C. Brunham, D.E. Low, M. Petric, R.L. Roper, P.J. Talbot, T. Tam and L. Babiuk, "Severe Acute Respiratory Syndrome (SARS): A Year in Review," *Annual Review of Medicine* 56 (2005):357-81.

[5]World Health Organization (WHO), "Epidemic and Pandemic Alert; Diseases: SARS." At www.who.int/csr/sars/en/index.html.

[6]CBC News Online, "In Depth: SARS. Severe Acute Respiratory Syndrome." At www.cbc.ca/news/background/sars/index.html.

[7]Thomas Abraham, *Twenty-First Century Plague: The Story of SARS* (Baltimore, MD: Johns Hopkins University Press, 2005).

[8]Henry E. Sigerist, *The Great Doctors: A Biographical History of Medicine* (Garden City, NY: Doubleday, 1933, 1958), pp. 53-54; Joseph Frank Payne, *Thomas Sydenham* (London: Fisher Unwin, 1900), p. 110.

[9]Jacalyn Duffin, "AIDS, Memory and the History of Medicine: Musings on the Canadian Response," *Genitourinary Medicine* 70, no. 1 (1994):64-69.

[10]Alfred W. Crosby, "Influenza," in *Cambridge World History of Human Disease,* ed. Kenneth F. Kiple (Cambridge: Cambridge University Press, 1993), pp. 807-11; A.H. Reid and J.K. Taubenberger, "The Origin of the 1918 Pandemic Influenza Virus: A Continuing Enigma," *Journal of General Virology* 84 (2003):2285-92.

[11]For a concise and readable history of this investigation, see Abraham, *Twenty-First Century Plague,* pp. 107-31.

[12]On pathocenosis, see Mirko D. Grmek, "Un concept nouveau: la pathocénose," in *La vie, les maladies, et l'histoire,* ed. L.L. Lambrichs (Paris: Seuil, 2001), pp. 29-33; Mirko D. Grmek, *History of AIDS: Emergence and Origin of a Modern Pandemic,* trans. Russell C. Maulitz and Jacalyn Duffin (Princeton, NJ: Princeton University Press, 1990), pp. 156-61.

[13]The full program and pictures can be found at http://meds.queensu.ca/medicine/histm/.

[14]The examination question appeared as follows:
"SARS AND HISTORY Question (10 marks)
This question is based on four different winning suggestions of Julie C., Vivian H., Kirk R., Becky W. – CONGRATULATIONS! PRIZES CAN BE COLLECTED AT THE HISTORY OF MEDICINE OFFICE. THANKS TO ALL OF THOSE WHO MADE SUGGESTIONS

(a) BRIEFLY describe any FIVE features of the SARS epidemic of 2003. Your answer may range from scientific to social aspects, and from outset to end. (2.5 marks)

(b) Connect (compare or contrast or relate) each of your five features of SARS to one or more different epidemics of the past. (7.5 marks)"

[15]A videotape of Dr. Young's complete keynote address resides in the Queen's University Archives.

Part I

MEMORY
TWO MEDICAL OFFICIALS RECALL SARS IN TORONTO

2

My Experience with SARS[1]

James G. Young

As provincial coroner and commissioner of public safety and security, my job is to pick the right people and then sit back and follow their advice. With SARS, we were able to draw on great minds from across Ontario and get them working as a team. Kingston played an important part in the SARS outbreak. Queen's professor Dick Zoutman led the Science Committee, and I often counted on him for advice. If you learn nothing else from what I tell you here, please remember that problem-solving is much easier when you surround yourself with good people and you are willing to listen to what they say.

Beyond the tragic deaths that it caused, SARS held important implications for public health. First of all, and like many other epidemics, it obviously could come back. The good news in 2004 seems to be that its virulence is not as great as it was in 2003, and activity in Asia had declined. Of course, now instead we have reports of avian flu; one worry is replaced with something that may be even more worrisome.

Second, the SARS epidemic was important because it represented a potential form of bio-terrorism. It definitely was not bio-terrorism; however, if you think of bio-terrorism as the willful introduction of a bug into a society, then SARS, like anthrax, could be made to play that role in a particularly insidious way. In contrast, it's really easy to identify a terrorist bombing. When I was walking down a street in Bali, I could tell where the bombs had been, even if I had not known in advance where to look. The problem with SARS is the problem with bio-terrorism in general: you are obliged to chase it after the fact, trying to figure out — not where it is now — but rather, where it has been.

And you must do this without the benefit of obvious destruction. That makes it much, much harder.

Third, SARS was important because in its early days, it resembled a pandemic, and we realized that we simply didn't know enough about it even to tell whether or not this was "the big one." It's easier now that we have learned something of SARS and what worked and what did not; but at the outset, we knew only that a new disease was spreading around the world, people were falling ill, and mortality was high, particularly in the elderly and workers within the health-care system.

Very quickly, we had to put together a multidisciplinary team that would try to change the mechanisms of health-care delivery. It succeeded because people pulled together to work, readily doing what was asked and raising questions later. Dean David Walker's group (Ontario Experts Panel on SARS and Infectious Disease Control), in which Dick Zoutman and I play a part, is now re-examining the outbreak and our reactions to it. We are asking: "What can we learn from that? How do we build a better system? And how do we build a system that will operate more easily in the future?" It's important that we make a careful retrospective analysis, but that's an exercise for now.[2] At the time of the outbreak, however, the exercise that was needed required people not to ask too many questions; rather they had to do what made the most sense and be prepared to study it afterwards.

Why did SARS come to Ontario? We got SARS because we were unfortunate. One of our citizens ended up in the Metropole Hotel of Hong Kong at the wrong time in February. SARS had already been smoldering in China for some months. A doctor involved with those cases visited the Metropole Hotel for a wedding. He turned out to be highly infectious at the time of his visit and he spread SARS widely: Vietnam, Singapore, Canada, Hong Kong, and Beijing all got SARS as a result. The first Canadian patient was a lady who stayed with her husband on the ninth floor of the hotel, the same floor as the doctor from Guangdong Province. She must have contacted SARS either in, or while waiting for, the elevator. Upon her return to Toronto, she was seen medically, but her health deteriorated and she died (on 5 March 2003). It was felt that her pneumonia was the result of an infection picked up on her recent travels and aggravated, in part, by her underlying medical problems. Nobody recognized that she had SARS, already a fatal new disease in China. SARS had not yet been announced to the world and it did not yet have a name. Her son soon fell ill and went to the hospital; after several hours in Emergency, he was put in isolation, but he deteriorated and died a few days later on 13 March. The first indication of SARS in the literature was on 12 March, the day before the son's death and long after his admission. Reports described a flu-like illness that was spreading through Asia with a predilection for health-care workers.

By 15 March, SARS had a name and a geographic locale: Asia and part of North America — that part of North America being Toronto. Unfortunately, the son of the first woman had spread the disease to some of their relatives and friends; and while he was in the Emergency Department, he had infected two people on nearby stretchers. They, in turn, spread it through the next group of people.

That ever-widening chain of contact is what posed our problem. By 26 March, we recognized that we had a provincial emergency, an outbreak of a newly named disease. But at that point in time, there was so much else that we did not know. We did not know that the cause was a coronavirus, although we assumed it was a virus. Having seen only two cases, we did not even know the range of symptoms; in fact, it was a week or more before we knew that diarrhea was a frequent symptom. Some people who presented to Emergency Departments with diarrhea were thought to have gastroenteritis; only later, did it turn out that they had had SARS. We did not know the duration of the incubation period. We did not know whether it was spread by droplet or by air. We had no reliable diagnostic test, no vaccine, and no treatment.

When we asked ourselves: "What *do* we have?" we turned to history. What would our predecessors have done one hundred years ago? They would have implemented strict infection control, including aggressive quarantine or isolation. Those were the only two things that were readily and logically available, and those were the things that we used. Did we know the characteristics of SARS and that it might be stoppable? No, we did not. And the worst of it was that we had to wait for 10 to 14 days to learn how the new disease would behave.

In discussions on 26 March, the first night of the declared emergency, we said "OK, we know there are cases in the Scarborough Grace Hospital. But should we assume they are in other hospitals?" The answer was "Yes," because we had been transferring many patients around the system. We asked: "Do we know to what hospitals patients had been transferred?" And the answer, of course, was "No." Furthermore, people may have come and gone from Emergency Departments, or they may have been visiting patients in one hospital and then gone into other hospitals. We had to assume that SARS was potentially affecting every hospital in the province, but it just had not shown up yet. And we did not know which hospitals would eventually be targeted. We had to assume that the cases seen that day were merely the tip of an iceberg and that what was visible then had started ten days ago, probably somewhere else. Not only did we reason backwards in time, we had to determine where the disease would appear in the next ten days.

As a result, we decided to effectively slow down the health-care system and to immediately put in place infection control at all the hospitals in Ontario. So we closed the hospitals to visitors. We carefully kept track of all transfers and restricted them wherever possible. We stopped all elective surgeries. We stopped elective admissions. We brought gowns and gloves and masks into all areas of the hospitals and taught people how to use them properly, because many had forgotten. And we used infection control aggressively.

We knew that cancelling surgeries put some patients at risk, but we also soon realized that, without this measure, we would be obliged to close hospitals altogether. Within a day, we had to close York Central Hospital, and by the time of the second outbreak, we had to close both North York General and St. John's Convalescent Hospitals. It takes months to re-start a hospital once it's been closed. Our decision weighed the risks of having to close many hospitals one after another against the risks of closing down the entire system for a few days, keeping it available for rapid re-opening as soon as possible afterwards. We also reasoned that this slowing down is done voluntarily and with apparent impunity every year at Christmas when we choose to stop elective surgery. That we seem to get away with it each December implied that we had a safe precedent. We made that decision and implemented it on the first night.

Our decisions were based on the best science available. Dr. Zoutman will, no doubt, at some point in your medical training, show you the way to make informed decisions based on evidence-based science. There's a hierarchy of five characteristics or confidence levels that you try to have in place in order to make an informed decision; for complete confidence, you want to have all five before you act. With SARS, we were barely at level one, but that was all that we had, so it was our best. And on that we based our decisions.

To recap, we had identified the index family and then the outbreak at the hospital. The course of the outbreak looks fairly straightforward now when it is shown on a graph (Figure 1). But we did not have such graphs as the one shown here, which was constructed retrospectively. We did not know who among many sick people really had SARS and who did not until three weeks later. By

Figure 1

Phase 1 and Phase 2 SARS Cases by Status in Ontario as of 14 July 2003

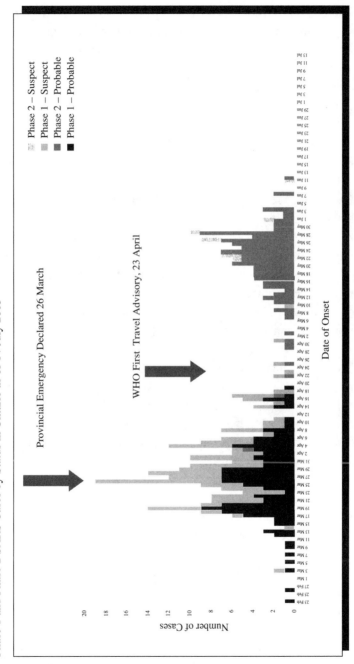

Note: Phase 1 cases are based on Health Canada case definitions prior to 29 May 2003. Phase 2 cases are based on revised Health Canada definitions effective 29 May 2003.

the second week of April we realized that the outbreak was coming under control. But a couple of days later we had to close two other hospitals, and we realized that it had spread into the community through a religious group. On Easter weekend (19 and 20 April), health-care workers at Sunnybrook Hospital were infected while doing a dangerous procedure involving the intubation of a SARS patient. And on 23 April 2003, the World Health Organization (WHO) decided we had a problem! We were a little upset that day.

The travel advisory instigated 23 April lasted until 30 April. It was reinstituted on 26 May and removed definitively on 2 July 2003. By convention, travel advisories are respected until twice the presumed incubation period has elapsed following the onset of the last reported case.

Counting twice ten days forward from 26 March when the Ontario-wide emergency was first declared, takes us to around Easter. Interestingly, the graph clearly shows the results achieved by rigorous implementation of old methods: strong infection control, coupled with isolation and quarantine of large numbers of people. Without understanding the characteristics of the disease, we had stopped it in that round. Perhaps, it was not neat and clean, and we still might learn a lot from imperfections in the experience, but it worked. It achieved what we had set out to do.

There was some spread of SARS into the community, where it had moderate viability. At the beginning, however, we had no idea how severe the community involvement would be. One case from each of the two waves, SARS I and SARS II, spread to the United States. Those events were sufficient to trigger the WHO travel advisory. We had to pay close attention to every single case, be it apparent or confirmed.

In all of this, we learned that our community cases could be tracked back to the Grace Hospital. Therefore, we could be safe in saying to Ontarians, "Carry on. Do your normal activities. Do what you need to do within the community." For the second wave, called SARS II, you see the same type of graph. We were already about halfway through that outbreak as shown on the graph, before we discovered that SARS was active again. This time we did not have to shut down the hospital system, because everyone already had gowns and masks and knew what to do. We just had to tell people to reinstate the methods that they had used before. If you count out ten days past that point, the wave of new cases is well past. In other words, things had changed greatly by the time of the second wave; we knew exactly what was needed to stop it.

The greatest challenge, in fact, was finding SARS in the first place. At the outset, we did not even know that SARS existed; and in the second wave, the small number of cases meant that it was difficult to notice. So the challenge of SARS, or of avian flu, or any pandemic or infectious disease, is finding it to begin with, before it spreads. Throughout your medical careers, you will hear a lot more about surveillance and you will practice far better infection control than we did for 30 years of my own career. Among its other lessons, SARS taught us the value of careful prevention, surveillance, and control.

NOTES

[1] This essay is excerpted from Dr. Young's speech, "Medicine and the Rest of the World" the 16th Annual Happening, 10 February 2004. The Queen's University Annual Hannah Happening is an autobiographical lecture for medical students delivered by a person who has made an important contribution to health care. Dr. Young's lecture provided the introductory keynote speech for the SARS and History symposium. His address ranged over many challenges of his career as Ontario provincial coroner, including his involvement with graduated licensing for young drivers, anti-smoking campaigns, the Swiss Air disaster, the attacks of 11 September 2001, the Bali bombings, and the Toronto SARS outbreak. Video-recordings of all the Hannah Happenings are available through the Queen's University Archives.

[2] The Walker Report was later released as *For The Public's Health: A Plan of Action,* Final Report of the Ontario Expert Panel on SARS and Infectious Disease Control (Dr. David Walker, chair) (Toronto: Ontario Ministry of Health and Long Term Care, 16 April 2004). At www.health.gov.on.ca/english/public/pub/ministry_reports/walker04/walker04_mn.html.

3

REMEMBERING SARS AND THE ONTARIO SARS SCIENTIFIC ADVISORY COMMITTEE

Dick Zoutman

I first learned of SARS while sitting at my computer sometime in early 2003. Almost every morning, I go to see what's hot by logging on to ProMed and checking the Global Electronic Reporting System. Hosted by the International Society for Infectious Disease, it is available in multiple languages to provide rapid notification of outbreaks around the world. As the SARS outbreak emerged in early 2003 and well before it had a name, I was aware that something had been happening in China.

The respiratory illness had been evolving in Asia from February or earlier and there may have been some cases in Canada. By mid-March, I was working on a plan for our local response at the Kingston General Hospital from an infection-control perspective.

At about 8:30 on the evening of Saturday, 29 March, I got a call from the commissioner of public safety, Jim Young. I knew him from his visit to Kingston five months earlier, in October 2002, for a meeting on bio-terrorism that I had chaired for the federal ministry, Health Canada. Jim announced that there was a problem and asked that I come to help. So on Sunday, 30 March, I was on the train to Toronto. I went directly to the building at 25 Grosvenor Street, which houses the office of the Ministry of Public Safety and Security.

The meeting of scientific advisors was already well underway in the board room of the minister of public security and safety, Bob Runciman. The room was poorly lit, almost dark, creating an ethereal, surreal atmosphere, and it was chaotic. People were huddled in corners, talking on cellphones trying to get information about what was going on. I remember Toronto microbiologist, Don Low, crouched down with his phone connected to a wall plug because he had burnt up his battery. Many sat with laptop computers, exchanging various versions of documents. Jim Young tried to corral everyone, but getting their attention was tough. I walked in on this scene as a complete newcomer, asking if somebody could tell me what was happening.

Don Low and Jim Young brought me up to speed with a snapshot of the situation: the numbers of affected people, and what measures were thought to be effective in treatment and prevention. Then together we had to determine a course of action that would fulfill our mission to advise Ontario's hospitals and citizens. There were so many unanswered questions. "What are we going to do? What do we want them to do? What kind of infection control was necessary? What do we do with the hospitals that had active cases? Should all the new, evolving cases go to one hospital or not?" Some of these questions have no simple answers. We agreed that we must try to limit exposure and protect certain hospitals. However, many hospitals already harboured SARS patients within their walls.

Then came bigger decisions. That first Sunday night we decided quickly to recommend a Code Orange alert provincewide. The ministry still had to mull over this proposal. On a nationally recognized system for various events, Code Orange signifies "mass casualty." It means you must stop elective care and start doing only one thing: dealing with the emergency. Patient transfers come to an end. It has huge implications for hospitals. Until then, I had not realized that a person can be admitted to one hospital in Toronto, have a CAT scan at another, and see a sub-specialist in a third. People had been shuttled around the city for different aspects of their investigations and care, and, of course, emergency rooms were hot spots.

Another big decision was to determine the criteria for quarantine. We made those recommendations without realizing that the same rules would soon affect those who were serving on the SARS Scientific Advisory Committee. Suddenly someone said "Wait a minute! Dr. Allison McGeer has been at Scarborough Grace Hospital and is now clinically unwell." We were mortified. One of our beloved colleagues probably had SARS, and it dawned on us that she had been with the Scientific Advisory Group on Saturday. All the committee members who had been there with Allison were exposed. The idea sent a chill down my spine. I thought, "I'm sitting here with all these colleagues. We've been on top of each other for hours, hovering over computers. Are they incubating an infection? Am I incubating it? Am I exposed?" It was self-worry: "What have I done to myself? What about my family?" But it was also a worry about everyone else in the province. If we are all sick, who will be left to do the work?

We had already approved the document for quarantine criteria, and now we were literally hoist by our own petard. The associate medical officer for Toronto Public Health, Dr. Bonnie Henry, had been heavily involved and in and out of the room; she was designated to evaluate those among us who were potentially exposed. This investigation went on late into the evening, well past midnight. Everyone met separately with her to determine their level of exposure; she had the authority to quarantine.

It seems ironic now. We were on the eighteenth floor and had sent the policy "upstairs" to the Operations Centre on the nineteenth floor. In the wee hours of the night, fatigue was setting in and I was madly typing on a computer trying to lay out the last details of the Code Orange and other guidelines for hospitals. One by one people went off to see Bonnie. Don Low returned saying, "Guess what? Five of us have been quarantined." But he reassured us that the rest would be alright if we had not been in the board room on Saturday: "You haven't been exposed," he said to me. And I thought, "Maybe he's right, but we don't know a lot about this disease. Maybe what we think is wrong." Self-worry again, the survival instinct was always there, lurking beneath the surface.

But the highest priority was yet another question: "Now what?" Before it had been created, the Scientific Committee already had new vacancies. Don Low said to me, "Good-bye. You're in charge." And to myself I said, "Yikes!" I know my way around Toronto in a very limited way: tourist spots and downtown. Jim Young decided that the committee was going to have to adjust to the people who remained, helped by others from across the province and the country. He said, "I dub you Chair." What was I going to say? The work had to carry on. So the next morning, everyone who was left gathered at 7 am.

I chaired what eventually became the Ontario SARS Scientific Advisory Committee (OSSAC) on behalf of and reporting to Dr. James (Jim) Young of the Ministry of Public Security and Safety. The committee was responsible for the science and policy part of the response. Operational issues were dealt with by another Ontario ministry, that of Health and Long Term Care. Inevitably, there was some overlap because it is difficult to do pure scientific policy without recognizing the practical implications of our recommendations. Whenever we recommended a course of action, we delivered it to Allison Stuart, director of the ministry of health and long term care. As a senior official in that ministry, she was in a good position to have her team examine our proposals to ensure that they would conform to law and work on a policy level. Based on their responses, we reworked our recommendations; generally, however, we quickly came to agreement.

The people who were quarantined — "the Q5" we called them — were all Torontonians who had had direct exposure to SARS. They included Don Low and the emergency specialist, Brian Schwartz, of the Toronto Emergency Service, who was deputy chair of the committee. I focused on the infection piece from a science perspective, while Brian, who had expertise in managing big emergencies, was more "macro" in orientation. Brian and I spent many hours working together and became good friends.

For the ten days of their quarantine, the Q5 were at home in their basements, dens, or laundry rooms — away from their families. We needed to hear from the quarantined committee members because they knew Toronto well. They communicated with us (and their families) by cellphone. I can only imagine how stressful that might have been. Some ordered fax machines to keep up with the documents. They also tried to participate on conference lines with only mixed success, considering the frequency, intensity, and duration of the calls. Occasionally we would forget to include them and they would be upset. Then an angry call would come through on another telephone line: "What is wrong with you guys?"

Throughout the crisis, the officials from both ministries (Health and Long Term Care and Public Safety and Security) were always helpful and quick to respond to our requests. They brought in multiple maps and pinned them to the wall. As our work evolved, we needed a structure, intellectually and physically. I sat at one end of a table that was so long that you could have bowled on it. At the other end of the room was a big white board on which we made a long list of things to be done and questions to be answered. Do we close certain hospitals? Do we recommend closing schools or other public places? We also made lists of smaller issues about an endless of array of things. When anybody touched the white board, I got very agitated because we could easily lose track of what was important. Eventually, we made a rule that no one but me should touch the white board.

Initially, only a few people were left at the committee table. We appealed to colleagues from Vancouver to St. John's. British Columbia's public health system is very well organized. Vancouver had seen a smaller SARS outbreak and valuable input came from Drs. William Bowie and Elizabeth Bryce of that city's Public Health. Others travelled from Nova Scotia (Dr. Joanne Langley), Saskatchewan (Dr. Alice Wong), and Manitoba (Dr. Joanne Embree); their outsider perspectives were useful too (see Table 1). We also asked for help in the form of an administrative assistant and a secretary. Again, the government responded quickly with Ruth Taylor Williams and Anna Amadouny and later, Anita Jacobson, all amazingly talented people who are capable of handling masses of information. Some of our committee members, eager to have reports from Hong Kong, were constantly checking Chinese newspapers online. We brought computers into the board room and asked to have the room wired for Internet use and fax machine. A horde of technicians attacked the room, ripped up the carpet, brought in ethernet connections and a fax machine. After two days, our operation space began to look like a machine with a logical way of doing business. It had become a war room.

Next we tried to devise an agenda, and chaos erupted all over again. We attempted to develop a system, but a torrent of items would threaten to take over. I would say "Stop. Wait a minute. We need to prioritize." But we were interrupted repeatedly. We would be deep into discussion, about, say, schools, do we close them? And what about the airport? But a phone would ring or somebody would bolt through the door, and the discussion would go off the rails.

So we established a *modus operandi*. At a desk in the foyer just outside our committee room door, sat a person who was instructed to admit only Jim Young, Allison Stuart, Dr. Colin D'Cunha (chief medical officer of health), Dr. Sheela Basrur (medical officer of health for Toronto), and a few select others. On the door was a big sign: "We are in session. Do not disturb." It worked. We operated like a court room: no cellphones, no "Blackberries," no "palm pilots" or other personal computing devices. We divided the issues and work among everyone. Beginning each morning at 7 am, we would list items in order of priority and then work at what needed to be done, disappear over lunch, work some more, and gather again at 4 pm to report on what we had accomplished.

TABLE 1

Ontario SARS Scientific Advisory Committee

The list of names of people who served changed over time. The following are those who served with me the longest, although not necessarily at the same time. All were volunteers and they worked under some of the most challenging circumstances imaginable.

Ms. Anne Bialachowski, Hamilton	Dr. Don Low, Toronto
Dr. William Bowie, Vancouver	Dr. Anne Matlow, Toronto
Dr. Elizabeth Bryce, Vancouver	Dr Allison McGeer, Toronto
Ms Sandra Callery, Toronto	Dr. Mike Murray, Barrie
Dr. Edward Ellis, Ottawa	Dr. Howard Njoo, Ottawa
Dr. Philip Ellison, Toronto	Mr. Milton O'Brodovitch, Toronto
Dr. Joanne Embree, Winnipeg	Dr. Aadu Pilt, Toronto
Dr. Ian Gemmill, Kingston	Dr. Virginia Roth, Ottawa
Dr. Bonnie Henry, Toronto	Dr. Brian Schwartz, Toronto
Dr. Ian Johnson, Toronto	Dr. Susan Tamblyn, Stratford
Dr. Gordon Jones, Kingston	Dr. Robin Williams, St. Catherines
Dr. Joanne Langley, Halifax	Dr. David White, Toronto
Dr. Gary Liss, Toronto	Dr. Alice Wong, Saskatoon

Unable to sleep, I usually arrived well before 7 am to go over the white board. I was one of only a handful of guests at the Delta Chelsea Inn. Toronto seemed empty: no tourists, few business people. It was eerie walking into the almost empty hotel, but the service was outstanding; they knew me by name and would ask "How's it going today?" The only sane moments in those days came on my walk from the Delta Chelsea Inn to Grosvenor Street. Spring was coming, the early morning air cleared my head and let me prepare quietly. I would look over the lists of things to do, read notes, sign the recommendations on which we'd agreed, and send them "upstairs" to the ministry. Then everybody would arrive, many at the same time.

It is easy to forget that we were all worried. Heads have to rule over hearts. You must tell yourself, "I haven't been exposed." I bought a thermometer to be able take my own temperature. In obeying the first rule of isolation and protection, we had security guards taking the temperature of everyone who entered the building. We understood the reason — after all it was our own policy — but the applications made us laugh. The guards were using tympanic membrane temperatures, and on those early spring mornings, we'd be as hypothermic as alligators: 32 degrees. We had to sign in and have our temperatures taken on the nineteenth floor, and then go down to our war room on the eighteenth floor. You could cheat by going directly to the eighteenth floor. But most cooperated out of loyalty to the project, and of course, we did not want anyone to contract SARS. We agreed that the committee members could not work in hospitals or be involved with SARS patients; otherwise we'd all be quarantined and no one would be left to do the work.

The operations centre staff brought in meals: breakfast, lunch, and supper, as well as coffee in huge urns. The food was often cool by the time we ate it. Under stress I ate — one cold, soggy French fry after another. Thus, I gained a ton of weight that I have had a hard time losing.

Eventually things settled into a rhythm. We would toil away on the issues of the day, meeting every morning with Jim Young and Colin D'Cunha to go over the priorities and pressure points. From my point of view, we had a fairly high level of autonomy to do our scientific work without interference in any way. The provincial Legislature was not in session; as a result, there was no Question Period driving us to provide answers for politicians.

We held midday meetings as an executive with Phil Hassen, deputy minister of health and long term care, and with many people from different government jurisdictions. How does it look to them, how did it look to us, and what are some of the things we have to solve together? Jim chaired those meetings. Sometimes they were tense. We thought we might run out of the N95 masks; which seemed to be disappearing into thin air. Buyers from the Ministry of Health and Long Term Care attempted to call suppliers hoping to direct or divert shipments to Ontario. We never ran out, thank goodness, but one of the buyers kept a graph. Showing us his curve, he said, "Deputy, by Thursday this week we run out." And everyone was horrified.

We suspected the cause of the disease was a virus because most transmissible respiratory infections are known to be viral. Severe bacterial diseases are relatively less transmissible, and that applies to most bacterial pneumonias with few exceptions. However, well after SARS, in an October 2005 outbreak in a Toronto nursing home, the pathogen turned out to be a bacteria, Legionella. This event was a harsh reminder of these exceptions. During SARS, virology labs were testing samples against all known viral pathogens. For a while, we thought it was human metapneumo virus which is a new respiratory virus first described in Holland. It was an intriguing hypothesis: a new virus behaving in interesting ways. But then reports came that it looked like a coronavirus. We were tempted to scoff, because usually those RNA viruses cause nothing more serious than the common cold. But veterinarians recognize coronaviruses as important pathogens that mutate through the animal kingdom. With this information, the outbreak began to make sense.

The media put their spin on events, both good and bad. We had real difficulty giving solid epidemiologic data in answer to their honest questions. There were issues around data not being as easy to come by as they should have been. We had no reliable mechanism for collection, especially in the beginning when no method could yet confirm which respiratory ailments were actually SARS.

Another aspect of the information problem was disease surveillance: we are a surveillance-poor country. Some days, I would pick up a newspaper at the hotel and read it on my morning walk to Grosvenor Street, because I could find stories there that I had not heard elsewhere.

Jim served as the spokesperson for us, because the media contact could have been all-consuming. He became the face of the outbreak as well as something of a movie star; he was good at it. I did only two media conferences. Each consumed most of a day, because there was a pre-conference, then the actual event, then a scrum and the post-conference. I was a fresh face and they tried to devour me. By the time the events were over, I was disconnected from what was happening back at the committee room. Normally I am comfortable with media appearances; during SARS, however, it was obvious that no one serving on the Scientific Advisory Committee should be doing them on a regular basis if we were to accomplish our other work. Subsequently, I did an interview with Ann Lukits for the *Kingston Whig Standard*, for which I obtained government consent. The government public relations people provided coaching, but they did not tell us what to say.

As for the jurisdictional confusion, it was clear that the public health division, under Dr. D'Cunha, had some worries about the role of our committee. It was confusion over who was in charge; to the Public Health Branch, we seemed to be an ad hoc, rag-tag bunch of self-assembled and so-called experts reporting to a different ministry in what was perceived to be a *health* emergency. In this case, however, it was Emergency Measures Ontario who provided the infrastructure for running things. We were reporting to both commissioners of Public Health and of Public Security and Safety, Dr. Colin D'Cunha and Dr. Jim Young.

The relationship with the Health side was difficult. Justice Archibald Campbell delved into that matter in his report. We tried to be supportive, we recognized that the commissioner of public health, who was also the chief medical officer of health, held a lot of legal responsibility and authority, as did his counterpart, Jim Young, as commissioner of public security. Indeed, any outbreak is a health matter, but it also affects all of society. Here again, over-lap is inevitable. Every disaster, earthquake, flood, environmental accident, would eventually have a health component. This health outbreak had a societal component that affected the entire province; for that reason it went to the Min-istry of Public Security and Safety, which already had an operations centre to coordinate the work, but was not provided with the resources to carry out the task. Even today, a large outbreak like this will likely escalate to a provincewide emergency as it did (and should have done) then. At that time, there was no equiva-lent emergency operations centre in the Ministry of Health and Long Term Care. In the aftermath of the SARS outbreak, an emergency planning centre was cre-ated, directed by Allison Stuart. She is charged with, among other things, building our infrastructure in preparation for an influenza pandemic.

We saw few politicians, which was encouraging for us. The minister of public safety and security, Bob Runciman, guaranteed whatever was needed to get the job done. On several occasions, we met with the minister of health and long term care, Tony Clement. Similarly interested and concerned, he also ex-pressed his willingness to answer to our needs. Ultimately, we let Jim Young deal with the internal government matters, just as he dealt with the media. He had such authority that he could go to a minister's office and say "These are the things we need." Most importantly, everyone in government knew him and trusted him.

Their trust was not misplaced. Jim Young has unique gifts: a good mind and superb organizational skills. He could prioritize well, triage appropriately, and he was comfortable with chaos. He does not take notes, he does not have a laptop computer, nor does he use e-mail. In the meetings, he focused on the issues and seemed to forget nothing. He also instilled confidence when things were looking awful. Jim kept us all together and he was able to act as interface between government and our group of scientists and physicians.

The worst moment (and I'll never forget it) was Easter weekend, 19–20 April. I had not been home in weeks. I wanted to see my family on the long weekend. I booked a ticket for an overnight train that left at 11:30 pm; I would be home by 2 am. I was so exhausted when I climbed on to the sleeper car that I was terrified of falling deeply asleep only to wake up in Montreal. So, trying not to sleep, I lay in a twilight zone, partially unaware, and I dreamt that Toronto and Kingston had been consumed with SARS and were desolate. It was the worst train ride that I have ever had. Half awake, I kept wondering if it was real or a horrible nightmare inflated by fatigue. I'd rouse and say to myself. "No, no, it is not really happening. Have a glass of water." Then I would lie back and drift into the same state — everybody was dead, the disease was out of control, Ontario was laid bare and I had failed, we had all failed. When the train finally stopped in Kingston, I was drenched in cold sweat.

The miserable journey was a premonition because the next two days were even worse. That Easter weekend the SARS outbreak seemed to deepen, in a fashion that we labelled "through precautions." In Sunnybrook and Mount Sinai Hospitals, two of the key sites that were handling many SARS patients, precautions were in place. Staff knew about wearing the N95 masks, gowns, and goggles and we had confidence that those precautions worked when they were properly applied. But now staff were showing up sick with SARS despite the use of these precautions; hence, "through precautions." We invented words and strange phrases as we went along. (The one phrase I really hate is "the new normal," so widely used and for so long afterwards, and it means nothing.)

But I was at home. I had not seen my wife, Heather, or my children, Andrew 18, Jeremy 15, and Cory 10; the absence had been stressful for us all. We spent a little time together, but I was exhausted and must have looked terrible. On Saturday the phone started ringing about two "through precautions" cases. I was using my cellphone with two batteries and a charger so I could change the battery; the phone grew so hot that I actually burnt my ear. There I was, sitting at our dining-room table, having these conversations, while my family was waiting for attention. In this profession you are always a little torn between work and family, but this was the worst. Though I was physically at home, I was simply unavailable. Trying to chair 20 people on a conference call is chaotic at best, and we were dealing with perplexing questions: Should we bring in the Centers for Disease Control (in Atlanta) to admit that protective measures are no longer working and we are losing control? All the while the horrible nightmare of the previous night was playing in the background. Coming home had been a mistake. Finally, on the Sunday morning, Heather said "It's nice having you home, but get out of here. Go do what you have to do."

Fortunately, nothing truly catastrophic was happening, but we didn't know that on the weekend. Soon we learned that the outbreak was not "through precautions." With fatigue and physical stress, caregivers were simply unable to maintain the high level of protection. It is understandable. Detailed evaluations to establish the cause were done and have been published since.

Another big worry was the Filipino Bukas-Loob Sa Diyos (BLD) community which had had a SARS death and a large funeral with the usual close contacts and many tears. The potential for exposure to body fluids made us worry that SARS would break out in that community. Until this time, SARS here in Canada was largely a hospital event. It never spread widely into the community because its transmission requires close contact. Toronto Public Health was quarantining people *en masse*. These actions have been criticized; however, there was little else to be done.

Finally, around mid-May we started packing up to go home. We had trashed Mr. Runciman's board room: marks on the walls, stains on the furniture, a torn carpet, and gravy from the chicken dinners on the floor. Knowing that there could be legal issues was anxiety-provoking. Soon the Campbell Commission, the Walker panel, and the Naylor enquiry were formed.

No sooner had we been home for a week when a second wave of SARS, called SARS II, occurred. It had a devastating effect on North York General Hospital. It closed, emptied all its beds, and a nurse died. During SARS II, we tried to work remotely by teleconference. We were all tired and desperate to be with our families, and working remotely went quite well. We made twice weekly trips to Toronto.

During SARS II, the World Health Organization (WHO) issued a travel advisory against visiting Toronto. It was a huge disappointment because it had no basis in science. The minister of health and long term care, together with Jim Young, Colin D'Cunha, and several others flew to Geneva where they argued that the travel advisory was inappropriate. But the WHO did not agree. The WHO officials later removed the travel advisory when the second wave of SARS was over.

As our operation was winding down, a new challenge arose: how to bring the health system back on line. When do hospitals re-open? When do screening measures stop? We developed criteria for when hospitals could open and graded them in terms of their level of SARS involvement. Bringing the system back was actually more difficult than bringing it down.

In the middle of SARS II, I went for ten days to a conference in Durban, South Africa, with Heather and my son Jeremy. We had booked long before with non-refundable tickets. I offered to cancel, but Jim Young and Brian Schwartz said "Go, you need to go." I felt terribly guilty. As we passed through all the airports, I was fascinated by their signs about SARS. We planned to go to the Drackensberg mountains and into Lesotho for a day trip, but no Canadians were allowed to make that trip because of SARS. Given my involvement with the outbreak, the decision seemed ironic, but I did not argue. There was no need for us to go to Lesotho; and instead we went for a guided hike in the mountains with ancient bushman caves and drawings and amazing wildlife.

As we worked on the scientific committee, we were constantly reminded of epidemics from history. We spent a lot of time talking about what we could learn from the 1918 influenza pandemic. We needed to go back to those public records and analyze the interventions used then. Unlike the people in 1918, we decided not to close movie theatres and schools, but those possibilities were debated in 2003. Our wholesale isolation of large cohorts of people in the community has already been criticized. If SARS were to occur again, we probably would avoid that measure because SARS did not spread into the community. But in the first outbreak, we just did not know what was possible. It may be argued that we overreacted and created a lot of work for ourselves. With fewer control measures and a more aggressive pathogen, however, the price could have been much higher. We erred on the side of caution.

With our modern technology, we are no safer from the dangerous onslaughts of nature than people were in the past. In some ways, this Toronto outbreak came about *because of* modern technology, including global travel. SARS started in Canada because somebody vomited in the hallway of the Metropole Hotel; had he made it to the hotel bathroom, maybe it would not have happened.

Near misses of potential new outbreaks could be happening constantly. At the time of writing, we worry about the H5N1 strain of avian flu, which is moving from Asia into Turkey and central Europe right now. We worry what it means and how global travel could make it worse.

On the other hand, technology has helped, especially global communications. Unlike the 1918 influenza, we knew what was going on around the world as it happened. But the rapid dissemination of information also excited the media and heightened the fear. Global communications also meant that the WHO could review our data on a Web site, just because it was there, and we know where that decision led. We wanted to be transparent and declare our situation; but the WHO came to a conclusion that was different from the one we thought was justified by using the same information. It had huge economic effects on Toronto. If we stopped everybody from travelling, we could probably reduce the potential for outbreaks; we certainly could contain them better. During SARS, as already mentioned, we had discussed closing airports. But we did not shut down air travel, and for SARS, it was the right thing. But will it be the right thing for another new pathogen? We simply do not know.

A Canadian team at the University of British Columbia, working with the federal laboratory in Winnipeg, sequenced the SARS virus. Their findings made a big difference to the biologists who seek to understand how the coronavirus could do this. Unique to the humanized strain was a 29-base-pair insert. Already a number of studies have examined the archeobiology of this insert. It may not have originated in civets and dogs, as was previously thought, but in a brown horseshoe bat in China. Bats are widespread and migratory and the bat strain bears a resemblance to the viral strain of some civets and raccoon dogs. A lot more work needs to be done. Coronaviruses are widespread in nature and RNA viruses in general are not very good at reproducing; they make a lot of mistakes resulting in mutations.

These discoveries are a fascinating, new science, but our methods of control were traditional. The US Marines say that policy is for amateurs, logistics is for professionals. Managing SARS was all logistics, with some intriguing implications. For example, at Easter, large church services were anticipated, and questions were raised about the sharing of communion cups. We met with religious leaders to go over the details and I remember one of the cardinals saying that absolution can be given *in absentia*. We all put our hands up to say that we needed it. The Church leaders were very obliging. In hindsight, it was all unnecessary, of course, in that now we know that the possibility of spreading SARS during a communion service is very unlikely.

One of the things that is a liability for us in infection control is "what-if-ing" ourselves into a corner. What if this? What if that? You can frighten yourself by counting how many drops of saliva come out of a speaking mouth; and how many in a cough, or a laugh, and how far do they travel? Eventually you have to stop and settle on the evidence, otherwise paralysis sets in.

When the next outbreak comes, we are somewhat safer. Since SARS and because of it, we have the Emergency Measures Unit in the Ontario Ministry of Health and Long Term Care. We have Dr. Basrur as the chief medical officer for the entire province, and we have the Provincial Infectious Disease Advisory Committee. We also have an entirely new federal agency, dealing with the old items under a new title.

At the provincial level, a lot of planning is being done, but make no mistake, we are not entirely ready yet. If we had a big outbreak, many important issues are still not resolved. We are more prepared than before SARS, but I worry about the information infrastructure. Around influenza, of course, there is *Tamiflu* medication and the urge to have large stocks. Even so, we will not have enough for every citizen, although some people think that we should try. Ideally, you need only one capsule a day for prophylaxis as far as we know. That's 35 million capsules a day, just for Canada, and 300 million capsules for the United States. The manufacturers cannot make it that quickly, nor could they produce that amount in a short time. At the time of writing (October 2005), they are limiting access to the drug to avoid hoarding. As a result, a triage list must be established to protect the most vulnerable people and front-line workers: who gets the drug and who does not.

If I have learned anything from this experience, it is that we remain vulnerable to pandemics. Our very best defence is a vaccine. However, that method was not possible for SARS and may not be possible or rapid enough for a new virus. Therefore, we must, as our second line of defence, be prepared for a pandemic. This action requires significant investment in planning for what we hope will never occur. An important part of this planning is conducting exercises. It is incredibly hard work. One has to view preparedness as an investment in our future and that of generations to come. To be caught unawares is unfortunate, but to be found unprepared when preparation was possible, is unforgivable.

Part II

HISTORY
HISTORIANS OF DISEASE REFLECT ON SARS

4

SARS AND PLAGUES PAST

Ann G. Carmichael

The SARS outbreak evoked different resonances with past plagues. The most obvious connections were immediate and personal, centring around impromptu quarantines and streets full of people in gauze masks. Health-care workers, who were at much greater risk of SARS infection than the general population of any affected area, also communicated their experiences with an immediacy reminiscent of Defoe's narrator in *A Journal of the Plague Year*, as they confronted the moral and professional dilemmas that their risk and fears presented. World Health Organization (WHO) interventions led to significant functional revision of international public health surveillance protocols, many of which were designed long ago with plague in mind.[1] Finally, evoking the past during the outbreak seemed to prompt later conferences focused on its lessons. Within a year, scientific conferences devoted to the SARS outbreak repeatedly summoned the image of "learning from SARS," an image that reso-nates with histories of plague written for medical and public health audiences.[2] Far from failing to remember the past, this epidemic led many to grasp such links both immediately and on later reflection.

Suppose the comparison were in reverse. What lessons might the SARS experience highlight within the long history of plague? Historical records of medieval and early modern plagues do not provide rich, diverse, simultaneous evidence from different participants, victims, and onlookers, such as those easily accessible about SARS. Records of past plagues are never detailed enough to allow a complete picture of how things actually happened, particularly in the first great history-altering pandemic. Of course, we cannot translate or fill in silences in historical records with modern experiences. But we value historical research and refinements to our understanding of history partly because, by enlarging our personal experiences, such inquiries help us to prepare for futures that we cannot predict and thus have not fully imagined.[3] If the past helps us to better imagine and understand the range of human experience, perhaps the range of human experience can now help to enrich our access to the past.

SARS IN CHINA: THE BEGINNINGS

SARS entered global history when 64-year old Dr. Liu Jianlun, a physician and professor of nephrology, stayed in the Hong Kong Metropole Hotel on 21 February 2003.[4] Some note with irony that he occupied room number 911, but global terrorism and impending war in Iraq were realistic fears during this time, and were easily linked to vague rumours of a novel epidemic spreading through southern China.[5] Coming from Zhongshan, Guangdong to attend a family wedding, Dr. Liu developed severe pneumonia and was admitted to the Kwong Wah Hospital on 22 February; he died there on 4 March 2003.[6] One of the individuals whom Dr. Liu infected at the hotel was a local resident, a young man called "Mr. C" in some SARS accounts; I will shortly return to his story.[7] Another was a 65-year-old American businessman who went to Hanoi, where he was seen by Dr. Carlo Urbani of the World Health Organization on 28 February. After being "evacuated back to Hong Kong," the businessman soon died. Urbani meanwhile recognized the danger, alerted the WHO offices in Geneva, and coined the acronym SARS for the man's cause of death. Urbani himself became the most noted victim of the outbreak, dying a month later in a hospital in Bangkok.[8] Two contact victims at the Metropole Hotel spread SARS to Canada. One was an older Canadian woman visiting Hong Kong, who returned to Toronto on 23 February, the other a man from Vancouver.[9] Finally, two of the three young women who brought the epidemic to Singapore hospitals were said to have stayed on this hotel floor that hapless night.[10] Early cases in Taiwan were imported from Hong Kong and southern China, but probably not via the Metropole hotel.[11]

Expert epidemiological investigations traced the paths of these individuals, typically looking forward toward the next people and places at risk so long as the outbreak was not yet under control. The advantage such communication and information networks provided is one of the striking differences between pestilences today and those plagues of pre-industrial Europe. Only the perception of an initial medical inability to control spread of the infection and to identify its microbial cause foreshortened the distance between past and present. Absent access to reliable information, the past re-emerged. What took place at the Prince of Wales Hospital in Hong Kong provides a good example of such a predicament.

The local Hong Kong resident staying in the Metropole Hotel (a 26-year-old airport worker) came to the Emergency Department of the Prince of Wales Hospital on 28 February, acutely febrile, with general malaise and myalgias.[12] He was treated and discharged because, being young, he was expected to recover, but he returned on 4 March with a high fever and cough. While he subsequently improved after seven days' intensive care, nothing about the case yet signaled atypical danger to those treating him. Naturally dismissing non-scientific popular rumours, and unfortunately lacking information then available to regional and national health ministries, staff of the Prince of Wales Hospital suddenly found themselves inside the outbreak.[13] Health-care workers began to fall ill, soon feeling that they were "at ground zero," of a lethal epidemic of unknown etiology and means of spread. Between 11 March and 25 March, the hospital admitted 138 individuals to intensive care isolation wards, 69 of whom (50 percent) were hospital staff.[14]

A human drama unfolded inside the stricken hospital.[15] On 10–11 March, the head of the Department of Medicine realized that there was a problem when five physicians in the Emergency Department, and eight physicians and seven nurses from the general wards were suddenly quite ill. Rumours circulated outside the hospital of a "doctor's plague." The night staff of the general ward assembled in the Emergency Department to undergo screening tests because the area had an independent ventilation source. When the illness of nurses, physicians, and support staff reached a critical mass, compromising the care of patients, senior physicians and administrators became alarmed, imposing aggressive infection-control measures within the hospital. Members of the senior medical staff, however, refused hospital admission and insisted on remaining at home with their families, meanwhile helping themselves to hospital medical supplies. Many of the hospital personnel were admitted for observation, but some (again, mostly senior staff) refused hospital care, wanting to be at home or at other facilities.

By 12 March, all staff with atypical pneumonia had to be compelled to remain in hospital. The hospital stayed open, because the Hong Kong Department of Health denied them the option of refusing new patients. Rumours nonetheless led to a 30 percent decline in hospital admissions within the week, and the hospital was closed to most non-SARS admissions. (The 12th of March was also the day when the WHO issued a global travel advisory about travel to and from south China.[16]) Those senior staff brave enough, or powerless enough, to remain in the hospital had what they called "council of war" meetings. Once a day all staff met in a spacious room and voiced their concerns, all wore masks at all times. Together they adopted an arbitrary three-week quarantine period, but their predicament steadily eroded their capacity to work efficiently on patient care. Remembering this interval, two physicians later emphasized "the social isolation: *being known as a worker at the Prince of Wales Hospital quickly became similar to being labeled with the plague.* Many staff chose to sleep separately from families and found no one wanted to talk with them."[17] [emphasis added]

Summing up these events: a very sick young man was examined and treated conscientiously with standard good care; atypically he did not improve, and so returned to the hospital, as he would have been instructed to do if this happened. Hospital administrators recognized an unusual problem only with accelerating staff absenteeism, during a period that coincided with the fitful recovery of the young man. The feeling of being inside a "plague," emerged when what was going on inside the hospital connected to rumours outside its walls: they were suddenly both alone and not alone. Their subsequent actions were governed by external events and internal choices, some of which were compelled by Hong Kong public health authorities, some by the reinvention of practices that allayed fear. They readied for war against the unseen enemy within, and they implemented various barrier-creating measures, some of which were determined by position and social status within the hospital. One group of doctors and nurses dubbed themselves the "Dirty Team" — masked, goggled, gloved, hatted, and gowned to do battle on the front lines.[18]

The story quickly leads to some other issues, including quarantine, but I want to pause it here and cast a backward glance to the early phase of the Black Death in 1347–48, to focus on those who dealt with the dying. Physicians in south China (and to some extent Toronto) were faced with a problem similar to that in the first six months of the Black Death in Europe: How do you recognize that there is something new causing illness and death? And even if you face something known and understood within medical science, when and how do you know that you are seeing the beginning of a rapidly widening epidemic? Once you know you are at the beginning of an epidemic, what then?

Within the eye of the storm, inevitably fear sets in. Second, health-care work-ers, individually and collectively, experienced the growing recognition that they were disproportionately at risk. Despite the routine use of many barrier technologies that both objectively and psychologically were supposed to insu-late them, they found themselves in harm's way.

This particular issue is one that deserves greater attention because those gaining immediate useful experience about an epidemic can be those most at risk. The incapacitation, illness, or death of first-responders creates a break in the accumulation of experience useful to those not yet affected. Regarding the Black Death, one commonplace assumption is that physicians knew too little to be of real help, and that the loss of trained physicians might have opened the door to new medical ideas and approaches.[19] Conversely, in SARS the race to understanding, cure, and prevention tended to exclude those with direct per-sonal experience, leaving them out of much of the later "learning" conversations.

What can be gleaned relevant to such questions from evidence recorded in or about the early phase of the Black Death? Rather than assume doctors and other caretakers were exceptionally vulnerable during the Black Death, as they clearly were in the SARS outbreak, we should look again at the evidence. Did, and if so how did, the Black Death pandemic lead to the next steps that Hong Kong physicians took when the full burden of their particular situation became clear? How do ordinary, understandable human behaviours both cre-ate and defeat control strategies to manage fear?

FOURTEENTH-CENTURY PLAGUE IN EUROPE: WHAT CAN WE KNOW OF ITS BEGINNINGS?

The great pestilence of 1347 to 1350, only much later called the Black Death, appeared with little advanced warning, even though several often-cited survivor accounts create a prehistory for the epidemic.[20] A physician commit-tee in Paris placed the epidemic within a context of astrological events; others emphasized connections to apocalyptical predictions.[21] The famous tale of corpses hurled into the trading port of Kaffa, terrorizing and infecting its resi-dents, and sending Genoese merchants fleeing for home, was recorded by a surviving lawyer five or six years after the plague had passed, a man who never witnessed the events in question.[22] Most of what we know about the Black Death was written months or years after the catastrophe, rather than at its onset, or in the midst of terror.[23] Some recent research, by Daniel Smail and by Shona Wray, offers valuable corrective to the common assumption that chaos and collapse must have ensued quickly. Wray shows that notaries in Bologna were steadfast and did not experience noticeably higher death rates than others facing the plague.[24] Smail shows that city governors in Marseilles responded calmly, replacing gravediggers as necessary, processing wills and testaments, though at one point the court had to move away from a growing stench of unburied bodies.[25] Florentines and Venetians likewise devised novel committees to supervise street cleaning, removing stenches that altered the quality of the air and thus rendered it more apt to become pestilential.[26] Thus, many assaulted in the early months seem to have assumed that aggressive efforts would counter the stronger-than-usual pestilence. In other words, the earliest communities and individuals to experience the Black Death (all bordered the Mediterranean) initially saw only that the plague was "atypical," requiring enhanced, but essentially normal interventions.

Jon Arrizabalaga's important work also emphasizes that physicians did not initially confront the epidemic with a sense of helplessness or mortal fear. Instead, they accepted familiar clinical and epidemiological frameworks for managing local health crises. For example, two prominent physicians wrote advice pamphlets for local civic leaders, explaining the basic management of public sanitation, allaying fears with the reassurance that the natural world was predictable and understandable through human reason. Both of these men — Jacme d'Agramont writing in Lerida (Aragon)[27] and Gentile da Foligno in Perugia (central Italy) — died soon after they finished their treatises. Another physician author, Dionisio Colle, lost his life in the pestilence, surviving until 1350 and thinking himself immune.[28] Astrologer Simon of Covino wrote from Liège that "the doctors fall dead, as really happened in Montpellier, where there was a very great supply of doctors, of whom scarcely one escaped."[29]

With few exceptions we must reconstruct reactions to the Black Death through the lens of survivor stories. The author of one of these, a Franciscan friar named Michele da Piazza wrote about Messina and Catania, two of the earliest-affected places in western Europe. Unlike Boccaccio's and Gabriel dei Mussis's more famous post-plague accounts, this memoir struggles to find a single clear story of what happened. Friar Michele recounts step-wise expansion of uncertainty, fear, and desperation proceeding to terror.[30] Often he asked, "What more is there to say?" only to recall some further story of possible significance. Collective reactions — scapegoating, abandoning loved ones, flight, and desperate attempts to summon supernatural aid — are often-cited features of this particular account. But the narrative is otherwise dominated by longstanding rivalries between two Sicilian cities, people bickering while being "delivered to oblivion."[31]

Priests and notaries became terribly afraid to serve the ill and dying, unable to meet the demand even if they did keep working. Notaries (drawing up wills that would ensure the continuity of property and status) and priests (unburdening the dying of the weight of their sins), were the natural first-responders to a mortality crisis at this time. Panic and/or high mortality among those first-responders possibly ignited the larger fire of general terror. But this is speculation: we do not know well the tipping points of terror even now.[32] Did street-level panic begin when people found medical recommendations futile? In contrast to religious explanations that could universalize the causes of catastrophic plague as part of God's plan or God's punishment for human sin, medical explanations played to how the natural world worked. Experience early on mocked and defied these medical recommendations even as medical help and comfort of any sort was increasingly difficult to find.[33]

To a limited extent, first-responders to the Black Death began to systematize personal barrier strategies between themselves and their plague-stricken patients. Numerous authors mention the vulnerability of those who attended the sick during the plague, and thus important medical advice focused on how to confront these personal risks. Tommaso del Garbo, a wealthy Florentine physician and Black Death survivor, gave confident advice about self-protection — although this passage was likely written after the epidemic subsided.

> Confessors, physicians, notaries, family, servants and others who tend to the *pestiferati*, before they enter the sickroom should open all the doors and windows, so that the air is renewed in the room. And they should bathe their hands, pulses, face, mouth and nostrils with vinegar and rosewater. And when they enter the room, they should have two or three garlic cloves in their mouths.

> And it is also good, prior to entering the sickroom, to eat two slices of bread soaked in good wine, to drink the remaining wine and to eat a few sweets or confections. When you leave the room, again cool yourself with vinegar and rosewater in the manner described, and keep a sponge soaked in vinegar always in your hand, using it frequently. Replace the garlic cloves with new ones.[34]

When physicians did examine a patient, they took the pulse at arm's length, turning away, refusing to look at the individual. Del Garbo counselled notaries to stand outside the sick man's door, and let him shout his last will and testament.[35] Another practitioner recommended blindfolding patients, so their venomous gaze could not infect the space before the caretaker's eyes.[36] The canon of the Cathedral in Trent himself recovered, but most of his assistant clerics died, and he began to notice whole families quickly succumbing: "and I say that because of these [events] that such a terror grew among the people that many of the wealthy fled to their villas with their entire families ... and of the monks and priests left in Trent for the care of souls I did not see any survive who had frequented the ill."[37]

When and why did panic unfold? We tend to assume that because so many people died and because "plague" denotes mortality without discrimination among potential victims, the initial supramortality among first-responders is just another example of plague's horrors. (The logic is circular: if plague, then indiscriminate mortality.) Excess mortality among first-responders of medieval and early modern plague cannot be demonstrated with available sources. Neither do we know if early mortality among them triggered collective panic and fear.

Likewise, emergency personal techniques in managing risk are usually assumed to be commonplace and commonsensical responses to fear in epidemics. But barrier technologies reassured medical caretakers and other first-responders that something could shelter them from dangers surrounding the plague-stricken; physically protecting oneself from pestilence was possible. By contrast, mere escape to the hills, woods, or wilds could not ensure protection. The emphasis thus shifted from explanatory models to pragmatic strategies, from understanding to acting. If he adopted mechanical barriers between himself and the stricken, the physician's positive social and professional identity was not erased when his medicines failed. Additionally, the ritualized and reassuring components of such methods are secularized ways of managing the fear of annihilation. So long as one had confidence that there was something one could do, terror or helpless resignation could be distanced. On the other hand, patients (and testators and those on their deathbeds) expecting one level of care and attention, could be terrorized by the unexpected imposition of interpersonal barriers.

Of course, fear and terror did overtake most communities from which we have detailed accounts, because the epidemic proved to be far outside ordinary experience and expectations.[38] The calmest voice in the eye of the storm was surely that of physician Gentile da Foligno, well-known in the academic world before the plague. Marshalling his courage in April 1348, as the epidemic gradually engulfed him, Gentile first published a practical *Consilium contra pestilentiam* for the local townspeople and for medical students overly prone to theoretical discussions. He believed his lived experience through an earlier pestilence would serve him. When he began to realize this plague was without precedent, he published two more advice texts. Before he died in mid-June, he was comparing the epidemic to the greatest known to him from antiquity.[39]

Flight also needed a rational approach, if it were to be successful in avoiding plague. Physician Mariano di Ser Jacopo of Siena, deflecting a lawyer's insistence that humans carried plague directly from one place to another, ventured that not everyone exposed to the plague died of it, and thus that prevention was possible. Those who fled to a (hopefully) healthier location, but still died of plague, had absorbed the toxic air before they fled, and thus the corruption of their humors had already begun.[40] His advice was to flee sooner, before the air became corrupted — a prevention strategy that would resonate with the logic behind the invention of passive quarantines in 1377.[41]

Even with technologically unsophisticated communications, the news of pestilence spread faster than the epidemic, which by comparison crept or seeped into each new niche. Eyewitness survivors uniformly describe the pestilence as a multi-month event. None of the populations to the north of the Mediterranean communities were in quite this same surprised condition as the geographically first stricken. Early on, communities and their physicians had to distinguish among all the illnesses and deaths that might evidence something new. Without such connections to rumours, it was possible to be in the same surprised state of those in Sicily in 1347. For many in the general public one may have heard of the Black Death before seeing it: many towns had to enact regulations to silence the ceaseless ringing of church bells for the dead. Venetians forbad religious groups their customary display of their dead on the streets, one of the ways mendicants solicited alms.[42] Thus, hearing the bells too often, or seeing too many bodies on the streets were clues about the invisible early presence of plague, if no rumoured warnings circulated. William Naphy and Andrew Spicer point out that even with experience, when people knew plague could occur, they still found it difficult to recognize its beginning phases.[43]

BACK TO SARS: THE RESPONSES OF ISOLATION AND BARRIERS

The SARS experience most recapitulated plague history in its reliance on quarantines, and in the reflections and studies of health-care workers who had to wrestle with unfamiliar fears and unwelcome isolation and stigmatization. Various barrier technologies that had been created in response to plagues in Europe, from 1348 to 1743, came to the foreground of SARS history. The present invoked the past. Because Fidler has analyzed the history and novel uses of international quarantine law in the SARS outbreak, I will not summarize that material anew.[44] Yet, beyond the logistics and legalities of quarantines lay the fears and reflections of health-care workers — a dimension of SARS that has other resonances to plague history. Physicians in plague rarely wrote about their own fears, and most nurses and paramedical workers in the past could not do so, because they were illiterate. Here the present informs the past.

The legacy of individually-used forms of barrier technologies from plague times included clothing, chemicals, and masks especially. Canadian investigators concluded that SARS was "contained, at least temporarily — not by the genomic revolution, not by advanced pharmaceuticals, but by old-fashioned public health measures like hand-washing, infection-control procedures, isolation of cases, and tracing and quarantine of contacts."[45] Surprisingly, risk management among those who cared for plague victims has not been well studied. Instead, the historical study of plague has focused on behaviours, information, and differential mortality at the community level. The burden of the SARS epidemic fell upon caretakers, in part a reflection of modern peacetime success in managing outbreaks of acute infectious disease. Most of the nosocomial victims of SARS, in Hong Kong and elsewhere, occurred among nurses and non-medical support staff (clerical workers but especially cleaning staff).[46] Did plague, like SARS, place health personnel at far greater risk? Our assumption is "yes," but we have mostly anecdotal evidence to the point.

One of the reasons that risks to health-care workers have not received sufficient study is that hospital workers have had access to technically more sophisticated equipment than patients and civilians could access. Disparate risks of infection within the health community are notable in the SARS epidemic. Outside hospital microcosms, general practitioners in Hong Kong were at high risk because they worked in districts of high prevalence. Eight of these primary care physicians died. Others relied mostly on "keeping a greater distance from their patients, spending less time with them, or avoiding physical examinations,"[47] a strategy that tends to undermine the routines of primary medical care. Even within hospital settings, clinical studies of the unique stresses on those caregivers at highest risk in an epidemic suggest that investigations on the topic were uncommon before the SARS outbreak, and previous work was frequently done within a context of bio-terrorism.[48] Retrospective psychological and psychiatric inquiries revealed that we know relatively little about these aspects of outbreak management. Retrospective epidemiological studies show that in general the risk of becoming infected migrated from medical and nursing professionals to the non-medical support staff of hospitals, who were much more poorly informed and trained in the mechanics of personal infection prevention.

Within the Prince of Wales Hospital, fault lines of risk were exacerbated by an odd quarantine imposed by the Hong Kong Department of Public Health, which initially did not allow the isolated hospital to refuse new patients. The staff divided into those who fended for themselves — including those who refused to abide by an in-hospital quarantine and went home or to other facilities — and those who collaborated to form control teams within the hospital. Emergency Department physicians Cameron and Rainer neatly summarize the benefits and drawbacks of quarantine on in-hospital medical and nursing leaders:

> The initial period of closure [of the hospital] was helpful in allowing the hospital to establish meticulous infection control procedures and train staff. Psychologically, it allowed staff time to manage their own emotions. Prolonged closure probably resulted in a negative effect because it prevented staff from helping the region to fight this epidemic as other hospitals became overwhelmed.[49]

Unable to help in the fight, but not fully responsible for the dispersal of disease to the community, Prince of Wales staff were nonetheless blamed (by colleagues at other hospitals) for negligence and substandard infection control.[50]

Personal success in confronting SARS depended upon one's level of education about the potential sources of danger and the ways of using these barriers to good effect.[51] Risk was shifted from the powerful to those who lacked power within medical hierarchies. Those quarantined outside hospital settings resembled the more vulnerable at-risk groups inside hospitals because they had difficulty following rigorous infection-control precautions within their homes.

They were told to wash their hands frequently, to wear masks when in the same room as other household members, not to share personal items (e.g., towels, drinking cups, or cutlery), and to sleep in separate rooms. In addition, they were instructed to measure their temperatures twice daily.... All respondents described a sense of isolation.[52]

Health-care providers and those who followed international media coverage of the epidemic heightened their own protective behaviours in the wake of the epidemic. News media meanwhile gloried in street scenes of gauze-masked shoppers. The international visual symbol of SARS and the isolation that it created was the face mask. General practitioners revised their clinical practices, adding goggles, gowns, robes, gloves and even caps to their patient-seeing attire. Many insisted that patients wear masks during consultations, and some even avoided physical examinations.[53] Two Toronto physicians, long familiar with infection-control practices, confessed their own translation of risk into the minutiae of personal control.

Handwashing was transformed from an irregular and absent-minded habit to a necessity carried out frequently and deliberately.... Seven steps in all, continued for at least 15 seconds, making sure that the thumb, the web spaces and the nails were not missed.... Better handwashing was obvious, but additional nuances became apparent. Wedding bands created a space where the SARS virus could hide, and so had to come off. But where to store a ring? One could loop it through watchbands, yet watches were also forbidden.... We no longer bit or shared our pens, and threw each one out at the end of every shift.... Shoes were simple, since we each kept a dedicated pair at work; socks were smuggled home and immediately placed in the washing machine.[54]

Thus, Drs. Schull and Redelmeier readily adjusted to daily changes in types of hospital masks, but noted that people at the corner store were notably uncomfortable seeing the red marks still visible on their faces. In addition to such mild stigmatization they mourned most the "loss of visual cues that normally inform conversations," especially in clinical and professional contexts. Patient confidentiality also became a casualty in the epidemic.

Psychiatrist Robert Maunder and colleagues at the Mount Sinai Hospital in Toronto translated these minutiae into a more formal study of epidemic-related stressors among health-care personnel.[55] Nurses involved in the epidemic's control also published studies on the stresses, predicaments, and coping strategies of those on the front lines.[56] Some hospitals did not permit nurses to refuse hazardous exposure to SARS patient care, even when they knew that hospital staff spread the infection.[57] Once governments were fully involved in the epidemic's management, some hospitals were not permitted to refuse SARS patients.[58] Hospital administrators resented nurses' demands for hazard pay or overtime compensation.[59] In most affected localities, medical and nursing personnel had difficulty complying with quarantine isolation until the second phase of the epidemic, that is, after global warnings had been issued and enforced.

Back to Plague: What Can We Know of the Responses, Isolation and Barriers?

Plague literature is often better focused on the psychological experiences of enduring and surviving plague than is plague history, which typically explains responses and changes over time. In contrast, plague literature typically invokes an "everyman" predicament, rather than the dilemmas of those disproportionately in harm's way, but it echoes the themes of isolation and a suspended life: a secular purgatory. From Boccaccio through Defoe, great plague literature emphasized the time and space of isolation as a journey toward redemption, either individual or collective, and many detailed and interesting recent plague histories use personal accounts, literature, and artistic production to examine what plague meant to those who suffered its ravages.[60] Modern secular societies lost connection to the spiritual opportunities that ordinary people once savoured in such interruption to routines, and thus the personal benefits of quarantine were left without literary space. In the modern world, quarantines have increasingly carried undesirable, politically untenable economic costs, and thus waned from medical practice.

Plague art on the other hand, particularly in the post-Reformation era of Catholic reforms, reflected the development of many tiers of hospital workers dedicated to the care of the plague-stricken. Enhancing the status of altruistic, non-stigmatized plague workers, plague saints offered strong positive depictions of St. Roch, whose legend and hagiography became exclusively connected to plague.[61] Roch is particularly important because legend held him to be a plague survivor who in life turned to the care of other plague victims. St. Sebastian, however, was more ambiguous, an Apollo-like saint who could both send plague and cure it. No part of his legend ascribed healing activities to him.[62] The reforms undertaken after the Council of Trent (1542–64) led to the elevation of many varieties of healing saints, providing models of dangerous medical and nursing care as a route to sanctity.[63] First among the new saints was Cardinal-Archbishop of Milan, Carlo Borromeo, who organized the spiritual care of the plague-stricken, both inside and outside the great lazaretto of Milan, and opposed the secular board of health by holding processions and other activities that ignored quarantine and isolation. San Carlo also clothed and fed poor plague survivors, but he engaged in no lower-level plague tasks. He thus became a saint modelling administrative roles during the plague. Instead, a different aristocratic ascetic of the same era, Luigi Gonzaga, carried the plague victims he found on the streets of Rome to a hospital commanded for plague use. Other saints, and even the archangel Michael, became associated with medical care to plague victims most directly in works of Baroque art.[64]

The strongest resonance that SARS made to the plague was the identity-distorting, silencing, literally de-facing mask. Interestingly, the Carnivalesque masks of plague doctors were not invented until sometime in the late sixteenth or early seventeenth centuries, during the period in which saintly, unflinching plague service was idealized in art. While advice manuals written by physicians at the time of the Black Death, as we have seen, described the use of vinegar-soaked sponges to filter the corrupted air around a caretaker's face, these early prescriptions invoked no special attire for the physician. By the late fifteenth century the conviction that the air around a plague sufferer was highly contaminated led doctors to advise consultations in open, well-aerated spaces. The robe with mask seems to have been invented over a century later than the interest in chemical barriers, but likely served also to identify those who had official sanction to be in the deserted streets. During plague, civic health bureaus typically imposed curfews to restrict public commerce.

Nameless second-tier caretakers of the later sixteenth century, individuals who increasingly formed the mainstay of patient care in times of pestilence, seem to have been at substantially increased risk of dying from plague. Occasionally, the risk was borne by the religious communities dedicated to dangerous service.[65] Many others, though we know very little about them, were pressed into service, were indentured by hospitals, or migrated in search of profits.[66] Those having to nurse the plague-stricken, rather than those writing treatises about the causes and management of the disease or those orchestrating public, population-level controls, most likely invented many commonplace, plague-associated barrier technologies, including the famous beaked mask and waxed robe. In the first published description of special plague attire, Rouen physician J. de Lamperière's *Trattato sulla peste* of 1620, the costume's use in Paris was acknowledged to be a version of the dress widely adopted in European lazarettos. Parisian physicians used an oiled linen robe worn over their clothing, and oiled their temples, mouth, and nostrils before examining a patient. They saturated their gloves with oil so that they could still feel the pulse. Finally, they carried a white staff.[67] The staff was used both to remove the protective garment and to signal to others their connection to plague; occasionally it was used to lift the clothes or bed coverings of a patient. French king Louis XIII's personal physician, Charles de Lorme, embellished the concept, by describing an analogy between the garment and soldiers' armour. His proud innovation was the adoption of Moroccan or Levantine leather in its construction, making it costly and, we can imagine, decidedly uncomfortable in the hot months of the plague. He used wax and added a "long nose ... useful in keeping the malignant air at greater distance."[68] By the plagues of the 1630s, physicians hired during the plague insisted on being supplied a robe and head mask, and some added requests or requirements for wooden clogs.

The costume was an extension of the development of barrier technologies that helped to create distances and boundaries between those who may have touched the plague and those who feared contamination. The gown and mask thus followed, rather than preceded, sixteenth-century elaboration of disinfection procedures and pest houses. But it isolated the physician from the patient and does not seem to have been used widely (i.e., outside pest houses) until the twentieth century. More often the mask in medicine was incorporated into medicine as a means of administering ether or chloroform, and, at the end of the nineteenth century, with surgical masks hoping to prevent the spread of infection from the surgeon to the patient.[69]

The link of plague to the mask was strongly associated with powerful images of a bird-beaked physician, but made little impact on medical literature until an internationally known episode in 1911. An older French colonial physician in east Asia, one Dr. Mesny, died during the pneumonic plague epidemic in Manchuria, 1910–11, because, it was said, he refused to wear a mask. As senior professor in the Peiyang Medical College and an ex-army surgeon, Mesny believed he would be appointed the chief investigator of the outbreak, and thus secure his professional fame. Instead, the Chinese district administrator appointed Wu Lien-Teh, a 30-year-old ethnic Chinese medical scientist who had been trained at Cambridge University. Dramatically, in an effort to disprove Wu's opinion on the necessity of masks, Mesny visited a plague ward, donning gloves, cap and overalls, but no mask. The third day after the visit he became ill and died, despite liberal doses of anti-plague serum.[70] Wu remembered that after Mesny's death,

> panic reigned everywhere, and perhaps for the first time in this period of two months, members of the public in all stations of life understood the true significance of this dreadful pest in their midst ... [and] the simple protective gauze-and-cotton masks began to make their appearance among the workers.... Perhaps during the panic the inhabitants showed undue precaution, in that almost everyone in the street was seen to wear one form of mask or another, though not all of them were worn in the proper way. Some of these masks were to be seen suspended loosely from the ears, while some were even worn around the necks like amulets ... [but] the simple gauze-and-cotton mask recommended by the Chinese anti-plague organisation soon became popular, and volunteers manufactured them by the thousands in their homes.[71]

Observations published by the International Plague Conference that took place in Mukden in April 1911, documented the distinct measure of protection that the mask offered.[72] Moreover, Wu, the conference chairman, had proven that failure to use the mask was irrational in an epidemic demonstrably spread by droplet infection. Nevertheless, the modern plague protection costume was not fully accepted until gas warfare on the western front, 1915–18, demonstrated the utility of the mask for general personal protection, and it would be needed and used everywhere in 1918. The mask as personal protection against plague — by which I mean an acute life-threatening mortality risk of uncertain provenance or nature — seems to have reconnected non-medical communities with this larger plague history with the discovery of HIV/AIDS and its fear-driven use (e.g., by police departments). Popular histories and documentaries of the 1918 influenza pandemic, widely dispersing early images of masked civilians seems to postdate the mid-1980s HIV/AIDS scares.[73] How and precisely when the gauze surgical mask re-entered the non-professional public space of the late twentieth century is a study I leave to others.

CONCLUSION

This chapter has highlighted some ways in which the SARS outbreak of 2003 helps to create new dialogue with past plague history, emphasizing the experience of providers and first-responders within the complex and various issues that plague raised long ago. We should not minimize the difficulties of perceiving the initial phases of an epidemic, for emerging infectious diseases are increasing in global experience. Secondly, we are (surprisingly) finally beginning to see the patterns of risk redistribution and the burdens on nurses and paramedical personnel. Here some new plague pasts might reinforce the importance of wider knowledge about their predicaments.

SARS was and is not plague. Even with new threats such as H5N1 (or "bird flu"), there is good reason to feel optimistic in the wake of SARS. While the Chinese Ministry of Health initially downplayed the extent and severity of a novel "atypical pneumonia" that appeared in Guangdong Province during the winter of 2002–03, the epidemiology and virology learned about SARS after early March 2003 could not have been pieced together fast enough to prevent its spread.[74] Scientists do not typically work from rumours. As it was, less than a year elapsed from emergence of the pathogen to its identification and control, an impressively short interval. There is similarly reason to feel lucky. Control was easier to effect because infected individuals became infectious when they became ill.[75] Had the virus spread only through respiratory droplet infection, it might have been suppressed even sooner. On the other hand, had it been possible to communicate SARS *before* one became noticeably unwell and febrile, a far more powerful global epidemic would have been likely, even with our sophisticated scientific surveillance and communication tools. The accelerating pace of emerging infectious diseases and antibiotic-resistant strains of widely dispersed pathogens suggests that we will need to harvest all the past and present lessons that we can to prevent the truly horrible die-offs of past plagues.[76] Finally, we might also feel grateful. In a larger epidemiological perspective, as well as from the perspective of plague history, the early efforts in management of a poorly understood epidemic among highly at-risk hospital personnel are insufficiently celebrated. Their actions recapitulate many of the practices of plague control, devised over centuries of European experience with plague.

NOTES

[1]David P. Fidler, *SARS: Governance and the Globalization of Disease* (Houndmills: Palgrave Macmillan, 2004).

[2]The most explicit examples of this point are: the Institute of Medicine (US) National Academy of Sciences, *Learning from SARS: Preparing for the Next Disease*

Outbreak (Washington, DC: National Academies Press, 2004); and the Public Health Agency of Canada's National Advisory Committee on SARS and Public Health, *Learning from SARS: Renewal of Public Health in Canada* (Ottawa: Health Canada, 2003), hereafter cited as "NAC, *Public Health in Canada.*" But also see the special issue edited by Robin A. Weiss and Angela R. McLean of *Philosophical Transactions of the Royal Society of London, B (Biological Sciences)* 359, no. 1447 (2004):1047-140, including papers delivered at their January 2004 conference: "Emerging Infections: What Have We Learnt from SARS?" Weiss and McLean title their conclusion, "What Have We Learnt from SARS?" pp. 1137-40; and Charles E-A Winslow, *The Conquest of Epidemic Diseases* (New York: Hafner, 1967[1943]), who dubbed plague "The Great Teacher." The recent "docu-drama" by David Wu, *"Plague City: SARS in Toronto"* [made for TV, 2005] suggests a further attempt to link plagues past with SARS.

[3]John Lewis Gaddis, *The Landscape of History: How Historians Map the Past* (New York and Oxford: Oxford University Press, 2002).

[4]On the illness of Dr. Liu Jianlun, see Keith Bradsher, "Hong Kong Faulted on Response to Illness," *New York Times,* 29 March 2003, p. 6: "The professor went to the Prince of Wales Hospital, told the staff that he was highly infectious and demanded that he be given a mask and put in an isolation ward behind double-sealed doors and with reduced air pressure to prevent any viral particles from leaking out. He then gave doctors a brief history of the illness before he became extremely sick." Elisabeth Rosenthal, "Confusion in China over Mystery Illness," *New York Times,* 28 March 2003, describes the abandoned hospital wards in Zhongshan where Dr. Liu had worked. Scientists, journalists, and sociologists have now developed an extensive prehistory of SARS, including some dramatic stories that pre-date Liu's ill-fated trip to Hong Kong. See Thomas Abraham, *Twenty-First Century Plague: The Story of SARS* (Hong Kong University Press, 2004; republished by Baltimore: Johns Hopkins University Press, 2005); NAS/IOM, *Learning from SARS;* Fidler, *SARS Governance*; Yanzhong Huang, "Epilogue: China's SARS Crisis," in *Mortal Peril: Public Health in China and Its Security Implications*, Health and Security Series Special Report No. 7 (Washington, DC: Chemical and Biological Arms Control Institute, 2003), pp. 65-77; and O. Wong, "Severe Acute Respiratory Syndrome (SARS)," *Occupational and Environmental Medicine* 61, no. 1 (January 2004):1e-3e. Electronic editorial at www.occenvmed.com.

[5]Not only were early cases of SARS occurring post-9/11, and in a season when many feared a crippling economic burden if this were another avian flu outbreak, many in southern China feared both their own government's cover-up and the US government's impending military invasion of Iraq: see, for example, Leu Siew Ying and Ernest Kong, "Whispers of War and a Spreading Influenza Outbreak Lead to Scenes of Panic Buying in Southern Regions: Rumours Spark the Great Salt Rush," *South China Morning Post* (Hong Kong), 14 February 2003. The *British Medical Journal* ran a story of panic in Guangzhou coinciding with an epidemic cluster on 11 February, at the World Trade Centre building, and concluded, wrongly, that this was only an "epidemic of rumours." Lesley Rosling and Mark Rosling, "Pneumonia Causes Panic in Guangdong Province," *British Medical Journal* 326 (February 2003):416. The

rumour concerning the World Trade Centre in Guanzhou appeared as early as 11 February 2003: Leu Siew Ying in Guangzhou and Ella Lee, "Panic Grips Guangdong as Mystery Pneumonia-like Virus Kills 6," *South China Morning Post* (Hong Kong).

[6]Several sources, including the *New York Times* accounts mentioned in note 4, mistakenly send Dr. Liu to the Prince of Wales Hospital. For a clarified account, see Abu Saleh Abdulla *et al.*, "Impacts of SARS on Health Care Systems and Strategies for Combating Future Outbreaks of Emerging Infectious Diseases," in *Learning from SARS*, pp. 83-87; or Abraham, *Twenty-First Century Plague*, pp. 63-66, who follows the stories of Metropole Hotel victims.

[7]Peter A. Cameron and Timothy H. Rainer, "Commentary," *Annals of Emergency Medicine* 42 (2003):113-16.

[8]Ivan Oransky, "Obituary: Carlo Urbani," *The Lancet* 361 (April 2003):1481. The patient actually was "evacuated back to Hong Kong," where he died on 12 March 2003. See B. Tomlinson and C. Cockram, "SARS: Experience at Prince of Wales Hospital, Hong Kong," *The Lancet* 361 (3 May 2003):1486.

[9]Monali Varia *et al.*, "Investigation of a Nosocomial Outbreak of Severe Acute Respiratory Syndrome (SARS) in Toronto, Canada," *Canadian Medical Association Journal* 169, no. 4 (19 August 2003):285-92. NAC, *Renewal of Public Health in Canada*, pp. 24ff, gives a fuller narrative account of the Toronto cases and on p. 26, briefly describes the successful arrest of SARS spread in British Columbia.

[10]Salma Khalik and Lee Hui Chieh, "Shopping Trip for 3 Turned Horribly Wrong – Women on Hong Kong Trip Brought Disease to Singapore," *The Straits Times* (Singapore), 18 March 2003.

[11]Po-Ren Hsueh *et al.*, "Patient Data, Early SARS Epidemic, Taiwan," *Emerging Infectious Diseases* 10, no. 3 (March 2004):489-93.

[12]Bradsher, "Hong Kong Faulted."

[13]Huang, *Mortal Peril*, pp. 65-68; *Learning from SARS*, *passim*; and Robert F. Breiman *et al.*, "Role of China in the Quest to Define and Control Severe Acute Respiratory Syndrome," *Emerging Infectious Diseases* 9, no. 9 (2003):1037-41, who blame "institutional interference" to the free flow of scientific information.

[14]Nelson Lee *et al.*, "A Major Outbreak of Severe Acute Respiratory Syndrome in Hong Kong," *New England Journal of Medicine* 348, no. 20 (15 May 2003):1986-94. Journalist Thomas Abraham, *Twenty-First Century Plague*, pp. 65-68 describes the hospital cluster with personal stories.

[15]See Cameron and Rainer, "Commentary." They provide the "ground zero" metaphor, p. 112.

[16]Fidler, *SARS Governance*, emphasizing that in taking this particular action the WHO broke legal and international precedents that were hundreds of years old. Fidler provides a summary version of this argument in the NAS/IOM, *Learning from SARS*, pp. 110-16.

[17]Cameron and Rainer, "Commentary," p. 115.

[18]O. Wong, "Severe Acute Respiratory Syndrome (SARS)," *Occupational and Environmental Medicine* 61, no. 1 (January 2004):1e-3e. Electronic editorial at

www.occenvmed.com. Nelson *et al.*, "A Major Outbreak of SARS in Hong Kong," instead refer to the brigade as "a team of *atypical pneumonia physicians.*"

[19]For example, see Robert Gottfried, *The Black Death* (New York: Free Press, 1983).

[20]Jon Arrizabalaga, "Facing the Black Death: Perceptions and Reactions of University Medical Practitioners," in *Practical Medicine from Salerno to the Black Death,* ed. Luis García-Ballester *et al.* (New York and Cambridge: Cambridge University Press, 1994), pp. 237-88, here pp. 242-43. Samuel K. Cohn, Jr. recently asserted that descriptions of the clinical features of victims during the Black Death do not offer any consensus about its symptoms. He denies that recurrent pestilence in later medieval Europe was due to modern bubonic plague, caused by *Yersinia pestis;* see Cohn's *The Black Death Transformed* (London: Arnold, 2002). Alfonso Corradi, *Annali delle epidemie occorse in Italia,* 5 volumes (repr. Bologna: Forni, 1972), Vol. 1, p. 189, n.1, and pp. 196-97, n. 3 almost as adamantly argues that the most common form of the pestilence of 1348 was bubonic, and the plague known to physicians' afterwards as *pestilenza dell'Anguinaja.* Insofar as Cohn also argues that the conflation of the Black Death and bacterial bubonic plague was made by medical scientists and historians at the beginning of the twentieth century, it is interesting to note that Corradi published his remarks in 1863. See also Salvatore de Renzi, *Storia della Medicina Italiana*, 5 vols. (1845, repr. Bologna: Forni, 1966), Vol. 2, pp. 294-306, Corradi's predecessor.

[21]Arrizabalaga, "Facing the Black Death"; Laura A. Smoller, "On Earthquakes, Hail, Frogs, and Geography: Plague and the Investigation of the Apocalypse in the Later Middle Ages," in *Last Things: Death and the Apocalypse in the Middle Ages,* ed. C.W. Bynum and P. Freedman (Philadelphia: University of Pennsylvania Press, 2000), pp. 156-87; Christian Rohr, "Man and Natural Disaster in the late Middle Ages: The Earthquake in Carinthia and Northern Italy on 25 January 1348 and its Perception," *Environment and History* 9 (2003):127-49.

[22]Gabriele dei Mussis of Piacenza, *Historia de Morbo,* trans. Rosemary Horrox, *The Black Death* (Manchester and New York: Manchester University Press, 1994), pp. 14-26.

[23]Similarly, later scientific investigations of coronaviruses and the socio-historical investigations of denial and cover-ups by Chinese health bureaucracies create a prehistory of the epidemic that could not have been seen so clearly as events were unfolding.

[24]Shona Kelly Wray, "*Speculum et exemplar:* The Notaries of Bologna During the Black Death," *Quellen und Forschungen aus italienischen Archiven und Bibliotheken* 81 (2001):200-28.

[25]Daniel Lord Smail, "Accommodating Plague in Medieval Marseille," *Continuity and Change* 11 (1996):11-41.

[26]Ann G. Carmichael, *Plague and the Poor in Renaissance Florence* (New York and Cambridge: Cambridge University Press, 1986); and Carlo M. Cipolla, *Public Health and the Medical Profession in the Renaissance* (New York and Cambridge: Cambridge University Press, 1976).

[27]"*Regiment de preservacio a epidimia o pestilencia e mortaldats: epistola de Maestre Jacme d'Agramont als honrats e discrets seynnors pahers e conseyll de la Ciutat de Leyda,* [Regimen of protection against epidemics or pestilence and mortality]," trans. M.L. Duran-Reynals and Charles-Edward Arthur Winslow, *Bulletin of the History of Medicine* 23(1949):57-89. The treatise's completion was dated 24 April 1348.

[28]Corradi, *Annali 1*, p. 185, n. 1: *Dei gratia ego immunis, cum fere extinctus ab hoc malo viderer, et innumeris remediis liberatus fui, quae exarare et communicare Civibus meis, et universes libenter volo.* And see Corradi, *Annali 4*, p. 36. Colle lived in Belluno, Italy.

[29]*De Judicio Solis* [1350], trans. Horrox, *The Black Death*, p. 167.

[30]Michele da Piazza, *Cronaca*, trans. by Horrox, *The Black Death*, pp. 35-41. While he described the events in a way that appears to reflect a spontaneous eyewitness testimony, he was in Catania, not Messina. The account ends with the deaths of the Duke and the Patriarch of Catania, to whom Michele is devoted, which occurred in April and September, respectively, 1348. Michele's remarks are part of his general history of Sicilia, 1337 to 1361. See Arturo Castiglioni, "I libri italiani della pestilenza," in *Il volto di Ippocrate: Istorie di medici e medicine d'altri tempi* (Milan: Società editrice Unitas, 1925), pp. 147-69, see p. 148.

[31]Horrox, *The Black Death*, pp. 25-26.

[32]Tom Pyszczynski, Sheldon Solomon and Jeff Greenberg, *In the Wake of 9/11: The Psychology of Terror* (Washington, DC: American Psychological Association, 2003) discuss some helpful recent research on the psychology of incipient terror and its management.

[33]Katherine Park's now classic study, *Doctors and Medicine in Early Renaissance Florence* (Princeton: Princeton University Press, 1985), shows that physicians lost social prestige and political power during the first century after the Black Death. Partly this happened because sons of prominent Florentine families stopped choosing careers in medicine, presumably because of the danger. But she also shows how the intellectual stature of medicine and physicians suffered from their inadequacies in treating the plague.

[34]B. Ferrari and S. Balossi, eds., "Consiglio contro la peste (da un manoscritto della Braidense)," *Scientia Veterum* (Pisa) 92 (1966):75-76. Also see John Henderson, "The Black Death in Florence: Medical and Communal Responses," in *Death in Towns: Urban Responses to the Dying and the Dead, 1000-1600,* ed. Steven Bassett (Leicester: Leicester University Press, 1992), pp. 136-50, esp. pp. 138-39. These procedures fit neatly within longstanding ways of protecting oneself from pestilence, chiefly by rectifying the air one breathed (even through pores, which were believed to participate in respiration). Here instead, I find the novelty lies in the elaboration of prophylactic rituals before a dangerous clinical encounter.

[35]Tommaso del Garbo, *Consiglio contro a pistolenza*, discussed in Corradi, *Annali 4*, pp. 43-44.

[36]Anonymous practitioner of Montpellier, translated by Horrox, *The Black Death*, pp. 182-84; on this treatise, see also Jon Arrizabalaga, "Facing the Black Death."

The danger that the patient's eyes presented relates to Galenic/Platonic *pneuma* theory of vision; see Rudolf E. Siegel, *Galen on Sense Perception* (New York: Karger, 1970), pp. 46-47. But the deadly gaze also resonates with medieval notions of the basilisk, which nearly disappeared from medical and scientific discussion after the anatomical revolution of the sixteenth century. On that topic, see Sergei Lobanov-Rostovsky, "Taming the basilisk," in *The Body in Parts: Fanatasies of Corporeality in Early Modern Europe,* ed. David Hillman and Carla Mazzio (New York: Routledge, 1997), pp. 195-217. On the medieval basilisk lore, see Laurence A. Breiner, "The Basilisk," in *Mythical and Fabulous Creatures: A Source Book and Research Guide,* ed. Malcom South (Westport, CT: Greenwood Press, 1987), pp. 113-22.

[37]Corradi, *Annali 1,* p. 197.

[38]For example, in 1457, a Florentine merchant, Giovanni Rucellai, fled to the countryside because plague was in the city. With time on his hands he went through old papers and found something his ancestor had written after the Black Death: "You couldn't find anyone willing to stay with the sick; and priests and friars refused to go to the sick to hear confessions or offer communion, because they said that the sickness would strike them.... The majority of physicians and surgeons died, and very few of them remained, similarly among the priests and friars few survived." See Francis W. Kent, "The Black Death of 1348 in Florence: A New Contemporary Account?" in *Renaissance Studies in Honor of Craig Hugh Smyth,* ed. Andrew Morrogh *et al.,* 2 vols. (Florence: Barbèra, 1985), Vol. I, pp. 117-28. There is one widely-cited denial of the onset of terror in the midst of plague: Richard W. Emery, "The Black Death of 1348 in Perpignan," *Speculum* 42 (1967):620-21. See also Darrel W. Amundsen, "Medical Deontology and Pestilential Disease in the Late Middle Ages," *Journal of the History of Medicine and Allied Sciences* 32 (1977):403-21.

[39]Arrizabalaga, "Facing the Black Death." Also see Lynn Thorndike, *A History of Magic and Experimental Science*, 8 vols. (New York and London: Columbia University Press, 1923-58), Vol. 3, pp. 241-46.

[40]Riccardo Simonini, "Il codice di Mariano di Ser Jacopo sopra *Rimedi alibi nel tempo di Pestilenza*," *Boll. Ist. Stor. Ital. dell'Arte Sanitaria* 9 (1929):161-69.

[41]Simonini, "Mariano di Ser Jacopo," p. 165. Mariano asks the recipient of this *consilium* to imagine a man named Peter (possibly a case the lawyer had previously raised). Peter and his friends become ill after fleeing to a safe retreat because they had breathed in the corrupted air of the dying before they left town, thus Peter didn't flee soon enough.

[42]Corradi, *Annali 4*, p. 37.

[43]William Naphy and Andrew Spicer, *The Black Death: a History of Plagues, 1345–1730* (Stroud, Gloucestershire: Tempus Publishing, 2000), p. 90.

[44]Fidler, *SARS Governance*; and see Fidler's earlier history, *International Law and Infectious Diseases* (Oxford: Clarendon Press, 1999). At the national and provincial levels, echoes of past *cordons sanitaires* sounded. Hong Kong authorities barricaded, taped, and sealed residents of the Amoy Gardens housing complex into a makeshift quarantine camp. Apoorva Mandavilli, "SARS Epidemic Unmasks Age-old

Quarantine Conundrum," *Nature Medicine* 9, no. 5 (May 2003):487; Abraham, *Twenty-First Century Plague*, pp. 68-69; and Tomlinson and Cockram, "Commentary: SARS." Mandavilli mentions that "when police arrived at the building, residents of more than half the apartments were missing and still remain at large." Hung, "The SARS Epidemic in Hong Kong" discusses the epidemic in the Amoy Gardens in some detail, but fails to mention this aspect of local government's SARS control.

General quarantine history in the wake of SARS was covered by Gian Franco Gensini, Magdi H. Yacoub and Andrea A. Conti, "The Concept of Quarantine in History: From Plague to SARS," *Journal of Infection* 49 (2004):257-61. Studies of earlier quarantine history include Paul J. Edelson, "Quarantine and Social Inequality," *Journal of the American Medical Association* 290, no. 21 (2003):2874; Howard Markel, *Quarantine! East European Jewish Immigrants and the New York City Epidemics of 1892* (Baltimore: the Johns Hopkins University Press, 1997), pp. 1-12; George Annas, "Bioterrorism, Public Health and Civil Liberties," *New England Journal of Medicine* 346, no. 17 (2002):1337-42; J.M. Colmers and D.M. Fox, "The Politics of Emergency Health Powers and the Isolation of Public Health," *American Journal of Public Health* 93 (2003):397-99; L.O. Gostin *et al.*, "The Model State Emergency Health Powers Act: Planning for and Response to Bioterrorism and Naturally Occurring Infectious Diseases," *Journal of the American Medical Association* 288 (2002):622-28; and Wendy E. Parmet, "AIDS and Quarantine: The Revival of an Archaic Doctrine," *Hofstra Law Review* 14 (1985):53-88.

[45]NAC, *Renewal of Public Health in Canada*, p. 42.

[46]J.T.F. Lau *et al.*, "SARS in Three Categories of Hospital Workers, Hong Kong," *Emerging Infectious Diseases* 10, no. 8 (August 2004). Accessed online at www.cdc.gov/ncidod/EID/vol10no8/04-0041.htm.

[47]W.C.W. Wong, A. Lee, K.K. Tsang and S.Y.S. Wong, "How Did General Practitioners Protect Themselves, their Family, and Staff During the SARS Epidemic in Hong Kong?" *Journal of Epidemiology and Community Health* 58 (2004):180-85. However, only 3 to 4 percent of all primary care practitioners in Hong Kong responded to the questionnaire, administered just after the quarantine was lifted.

[48]Robert Maunder *et al.*, "The Immediate Psychological and Occupational Impact of the 2003 SARS Outbreak in a Teaching Hospital," *Canadian Medical Association Journal* 168, no. 10 (13 May 2003):1245-51; and R. Maunder, "The Experience of the 2003 SARS Outbreak as a Traumatic Stress among Frontline Healthcare Workers in Toronto: Lessons Learned," *Philosophical Transactions of the Royal Society of London, B* 359 (2004):1117-25.

[49]Cameron and Rainer, "Commentary," p. 115.

[50]Abraham, *Twenty-First Century Plague*, pp. 68-69. See also Tomlinson and Cockram, "Commentary: SARS." Because the Prince of Wales Hospital was still "open," a patient returning to the Amoy Gardens sparked the dramatic, localized outbreak among residents of a large housing complex. Epidemiological analysis of these cases led to the important conclusion that SARS was not spread by droplet infection alone.

[51]It also depended upon where one was in the information food-chain. Simply Google "SARS nurses" to obtain a sense of how late and how selectively the primary patient-care individuals were provided up-to-date information about the unfolding epidemic.

[52]Hawrluck, "SARS Control," pp. 1206 and 1210. Many individual stories of lives in quarantine can be found in the *Toronto Star* in April 2003. Absence of official recommendations invited Hong Kong citizens to invent their own procedures and rationales for personal safety. See Joseph T.F. Liu *et al.*, "SARS-related Perceptions in Hong Kong," *Emerging Infectious Diseases* 11, no. 3 (March 2005):417-24. See also the summary provided by the NAC, *Renewal of Public Health in Canada*, pp. 41-42.

[53]Wong *et al.*, "General Practitioners;" Lau *et al.*, "SARS in Three Categories."

[54]Michael J Schull and Donald A Redelmeier, "Infection Control for the Dis-interested," *Canadian Medical Association Journal* 169, no. 2 (2003):122-23.

[55]Maunder *et al.*, "Immediate Impact;" and Maunder, "Experience of the 2003 SARS Outbreak."

[56]Betty Pui Man Chung *et al.*, "SARS: Caring for Patients in Hong Kong," *Journal of Clinical Nursing* 14 (2005):510-17; Sophia S.C. Chan *et al.*, "The Impact of Work-related Risk on Nurses during the SARS Outbreak in Hong Kong," *Family Community Health* 28, no. 3 (2005):274-87.

[57]Dyanne D. Affonso, Gavin J. Andrews and Lianne Jeffs, "The Urban Geog-raphy of SARS: Paradoxes and Dilemmas in Toronto's Health Care," *Journal of Advanced Nursing* 45, no. 6 (2004):568-78; Donald McNeil, "SARS Fears Spark Walkout by Health Workers in Taiwan," *The Age*, 21 May 2003. At www.theage.com.au/articles/2003/05/21/1053196639992.html.

[58]C. David Naylor, Cyril Chantler and Sian Griffiths, "Learning from SARS in Hong Kong and Toronto," *Journal of the American Medical Association* 291, no. 20 (2004):2483-87.

[59]NAC, *Renewal of Public Health in Canada*, p. 42.

[60]For two recent examples, see A. Lloyd Moote and Dorothy C. Moote, *The Great Plague: The Story of London's Most Deadly Year* (Baltimore: the Johns Hopkins University Press, 2004); and Gauvin A. Bailey, Pamela M. Jones, Franco Mormando and Thomas Worcester, eds., *Hope and Healing: Painting in Italy in a Time of Plague, 1500-1800* (Worcester, MA: Clark University College of the Holy Cross, and the Worcester Art Museum, distributed by the University of Chicago Press, 2005).

[61]Thomas Worcester, "St. Roch vs. Plague, Famine, and Fear," in *Hope and Healing: Painting in Italy in a Time of Plague, 1500-1800,* ed. Gauvin A. Bailey *et al.* (Worcester, MA: Worcester Art Museum, College of the Holy Cross; distributed by University of Chicago Press, 2005), pp. 153-76. All the essays in this volume relate to the general theme of Reformation-era Catholic art and literature. See also the brief, but useful, Donatella Lippe and Andrea A. Conti, "Plague, Policy, Saints and Terror-ists: A Historical Survey," 44, no. 4 (2002):226-28.

[62]Francesco Mormando, "Introduction: Response to the Plague in Early Mod-ern Italy: What the Primary Sources, Printed and Painted, Reveal," in *Hope and Healing,*

pp. 30-32; and Sheila C. Barker, "Plague Art in Early Modern Rome: Divine Directives and Temporal Remedies," in *Hope and Healing*, p. 48.

[63]Pamela M. Jones, "San Carlo Borromeo and Plague Imagery in Milan and Rome," in *Hope and Healing*, p. 66. In general, see the collection edited and introduced by Ole Peter Grell, Andrew Cunningham and Jon Arrizabalaga, *Health Care and Poor Relief in Counter-Reformation Europe* (London and New York: Routledge, 1999).

[64]For examples, Pope Gregory the Great (from his associations with the plague of 590 in Rome); Camillo of Lellis (founder of a healing order); Filippo Neri (a Jesuit devoted to hospital service); John of God (whose Hospitaller devotees in Rome led to his association with plague); and even Anthony of Padua (more usually associated with "St. Anthony's Fire"). See also Christine M. Boeckl, "Images of Plague and Pestilence," in *Sixteenth-Century Essays and Studies*, Vol. 53 (Kirksville, MO: Truman State University Press, 2000), pp. 55-60.

[65]Two essays in *Health Care and Poor Relief in Counter-Reformation Europe* allude to high mortality among religious devotees working in plague settings: David Gentilcore, "Cradle of Saints and Useful Institutions: Health Care and Poor Relief in the Kingdom of Naples," pp. 132-150; and Silvia Da Renzi, "A Fountain for the Thirsty and a Bank for the Pope: Charity, Conflicts, and Medical Careers at the Hospital of Santo Spirito in Seventeenth-Century Rome," pp. 102-31.

[66]William Naphy, *Plagues, Poisons and Potions: Plague-Spreading Conspiracies in the Western Alps, c.* 1530-1640 (Manchester and New York: Manchester University Press, 2002), follows the inquisitorial trials of lazaretto personnel who were not serving for the sake of their souls or love of the poor. Many were accused of spreading plague.

[67]Jacqueline Brossollet, Richard J. Palmer and Andreina Zitelli provide details to accompany illustrations, in the exhibit catalogue, *Venezia e la peste, 1348/1797*, Comune di Venezia, 2nd edition (Venice: Marsilio, 1980), pp. 63-70.

[68]As quoted in ibid., p. 65, my translation. Also see Carlo Cipolla, *Fighting the Plague in Seventeenth-Century Italy* (Madison, WI: University of Wisconsin Press, 1981), pp. 9-14. Surviving masks of the early nineteenth century are illustrated in Naphy and Spicer, *Black Death*, p. 165.

[69]Roy Porter, *The Greatest Benefit to Mankind* (New York: Norton, 1997), pp. 373-74.

[70]Lien-Teh Wu, *Plague Fighter: The Autobiography of a Modern Chinese Physician* (Cambridge: Heffer, 1960), pp. 19-21. Wu and his assistants were staying in the Hotel Metropole in Harbin!

[71]Ibid., pp. 21-22.

[72]John Gerlitt, "The Development of Quarantine," *Ciba Symposia* 2, no. 6 (1940):566-80, provides numerous illustrations of anti-plague masks, including one used in the Manchuria epidemic, but no discussion of their development.

[73]Alfred Crosby's publication, *America's Forgotten Pandemic: The Influenza of 1918,* (Cambridge: Cambridge University Press, 1989, with a second edition in

2003), was initially published as *Epidemic and Peace: 1918*, in 1976, coinciding with furor over the swine flu vaccination debacle. In citing both the re-publication and the second edition of this valuable book, I am arguing that return to the lessons and images of 1918 personal-barrier technologies came after public focus on masks as a means of protecting oneself against HIV/AIDS. Routine use of masks in hospitals between 1918–19 and the 1980s thus seems to me to centre around protection of patients — those undergoing surgical procedures, those with extensive burns, or those who were immunosuppressed and thus highly vulnerable.

[74]Yanzhou Huang, "The SARS Epidemic and its Aftermath in China: A Political Perspective," in *Learning from SARS*, pp. 116-36. But see also Ho-Fung Hung, "The Politics of SARS: Containing the Perils of Globalization by more Globalization," *Asian Perspective* 28, no. 1 (2004):19-44. Hung shows that idealized international controls to some extent reflected longstanding attitudes of "yellow peril," accentuating the ways in which Chinese public health officials drew criticism.

[75]J.S.M. Peiris and Y. Guan, "Confronting SARS: A View from Hong Kong," *Philosophical Transactions of the Royal Society of London, B* 359 (2004):1075-79.

[76]A.J. McMichael, "Environmental and Social Influences on Emerging Infectious Diseases: Past, Present and Future," *Philosophical Transactions of the Royal Society of London, B* 359 (2004):1049-58.

5

SARS Viewed from the Etiological Standpoint

K. Codell Carter

S ARS came along at a moment in time when the idea that an infectious disease must have a single, unique cause had already captured the scientific and popular imagination. We can contrast its arrival with the multi-factorial possibilities that greeted new infectious problems in a fairly recent past, obscuring solutions that seem obvious to us now. Individual patients with the same disease could have personalized reasons for being ill and vastly different needs for treatment. In this chapter, the rise of etiological thinking will be traced with reference to its many successes, including SARS. Each triumph served to consolidate this thinking as science. But conditions, such as cancer, that have yet to find unique causes, remind us to consider the etiological possibilities (and impossibilities) that are virtually invisible to us now because of our temporal commitment to the notion of a single, unique cause.

In 1845, Wilhelm Friedrich Scanzoni, director of the Prague maternity clinic, outlined a proposal for a study of the etiology of childbed fever. He recommended, in part, requiring local physicians to report the cause of each case of the disease in their practices.[1] Scanzoni's idea was that by tabulating these results one could determine, once and for all, the most prevalent causes of this dreaded disease. Medical texts from the early nineteenth century contain the results of surveys such as the one Scanzoni proposed. For example, in 1842, A.F. Chomel, a leading French internist, reported that he had investigated the causes of pneumonia "by interrogating carefully [75] individuals

struck by this affliction, and by directing ... questions to the causes that produced it"[2] Fourteen patients reported experiencing some form of cooling, five
had consumed too much wine, two had worked excessively, and another had
inhaled carbon vapor; the remaining 56 patients were unable to explain how
they had become ill.

Similar lists of causes can be found for nearly every disease in virtually
every medical text written in English, French, or German in the first half of the
nineteenth century. For example, in an 1845 medical text, James L. Bardsley, a
respected British physician, listed the following possible causes of diabetes:
frequent exposure to sudden alterations of heat and cold, indulgence in large
draughts of cold fluids when the system has been overheated by exercise, in-
temperate use of spirituous liquors, poor living, sleeping out the whole of the
night in a state of intoxication, checking perspiration suddenly, and mental
anxiety and distress.[3]

If a disease is defined as a collection of symptoms, virtually every disease will have, must have, a variety of unrelated causes, and, in the early
nineteenth century, diseases were almost always defined in terms of symptoms. For example, in one 1830 publication, hydrophobia, now generally called
rabies, was defined as an aversion to liquids so intense that swallowing was
impossible.[4] Writers in the period observed, correctly, that this condition could
be caused by blows to the throat or by psychological disorders as well as by
the bites of rabid animals. Thus, if diseases are defined in terms of symptoms,
since the same physical symptoms can come about in different ways, one
inevitably ends up with lists of possible causes, some more plausible than others,
as we have seen illustrated in the previous paragraph.

Obviously, physicians in this period thought about causes quite differently from how most physicians think today. What sorts of causes were of
interest to physicians in the early nineteenth century? In this context I can only
summarize what I have explained and documented elsewhere.[5] First, in the
early nineteenth century, physicians were interested in explaining why each
individual patient became ill, not in identifying what we would now think of
as *the* cause of some disease. Second, as a result, the causes they identified
were almost exclusively understood to be *sufficient* causes for *particular instances* of illness.[6] By contrast, today, we generally talk about *the* cause of
some disease, and we are almost exclusively concerned with a *necessary* cause
that is universal in the sense of being *common to all instances* of that disease.

Third, while at first glance it may seem difficult to understand what function the earlier way of thinking could have served, in fact it was part of a reasonable, coherent, and remarkably tenacious system of thought that had enormous social utility.

However, while focusing on causes of individual cases of illness served certain purposes and was reasonable, in retrospect it had two major deficiencies. First, if each disease is so construed as to have a variety of different causes, different cases of the same one disease will require entirely different treatments and a wide range of unrelated preventative measures. Indeed, nineteenth-century physicians cheerfully acknowledged that different cases of the very same disease could require diametrically opposed treatments. Because of this, diagnosis had little to do with choice of treatment, and systematic treatment and prophylaxis were virtually impossible. Second, because one usually explains the world in terms of causes, coherent explanations of disease phenomena were also impossible. If different cases of a given disease stem from unrelated causes, there must be different explanations of disease phenomena even for different cases of the same disease.

In this confused and confusing situation, medicine could be practised as an art, but scientific medicine, as we know it, was impossible. So far as one can determine from the historical and anthropological literature, this way of thinking dominated all of medicine throughout history and throughout the entire world until about the middle of the nineteenth century. In Europe, things then began to change.

In 1844, Jacob Henle published an essay vigorously criticizing contemporary medical thinking about causes.[7] According to Henle, typical etiological discussions were so fallacious that medicine appeared ridiculous in comparison to the exact sciences. He called for the identification of universal causes of diseases that were both necessary and sufficient. In fact, between about 1835 and 1850 several researchers identified causes of the sort that Henle seems to have had in mind. The earliest examples all appeared at about the same time, but they seem not to have been related in any way and they involved a range of different diseases. In 1835, an Italian student named Renucci persuaded the French medical establishment that scabies or itch was invariably due to minute but just barely visible acares mites.[8] In the same year, as a result of inoculation experiments on his own patients, Philippe Ricord became convinced that syphilis could only be induced by exposure to what he called "a special ferment" originating in existing syphilitic infections.[9] Also in 1835, Augustino Bassi published a book arguing that muscardine, a disease of silk worms, was always caused by a minute fungus.[10] In the early 1840s, David Gruby, a Hungarian microscopist, demonstrated that several skin diseases were also due to minute fungi.[11] Beginning in 1847, Ignaz Semmelweis argued that every case of childbed fever — puerperal sepsis — was due to the resorption of decaying organic matter.[12]

How did these discoveries come about? Greatly simplifying the histories, given a symptomatically defined disease, by using tests more or less like those later codified in Koch's Postulates,[13] researchers identified a cause that was sometimes sufficient for the onset of those symptoms. Either consciously or not, the disease was then redefined in terms of that cause. The new definition made each cause *universal* (one holding for every case of the disease) and *necessary* (one without which the disease could not occur). Why do we care about universal causes? Because given a universal cause, it is possible to formulate explanations that will hold in every case of a given disease. Why do we care about necessary causes? Because by avoiding a necessary cause, one avoids the effect. Since, in dealing with disease, one is usually interested in avoiding certain effects, namely the diseases in question, if possible, one wants to identify causes that are necessary.

A crucial step in the process of making causes universal and necessary is redefining the disease in terms of a cause. If one conceives of some disease as a collection of symptoms, in general the disease will not have a universal and necessary cause. Of course, on one level, such a redefinition could be seen as a mere verbal trick, a matter of semantics, and at the time, some of the new definitions were dismissed in just this way. For example, redefining syphilis in terms of a special ferment still left, unexplained and outside potential control, many symptomatically identical cases that had previously been called syphilis but were now *by definition* excluded from consideration. To critics, this seemed like removing a problem by defining it away, and one physician actually referred to one use of this approach as an "Egg of Columbus."[14] But remarkably, the change was precisely what was required to create scientific medicine. Antoine Lavoisier, the great French chemist, wrote that: "we cannot improve the language of any science without at the same time improving the science itself; neither can we, on the other hand, improve a science without improving its nomenclature."[15] What happened in medicine beginning about 1835 is a perfect and striking example. By 1880, in place of the lists of unrelated causes previously given for virtually every disease, one finds the assumption that each disease can be conceived as having a single, unique cause if only one can find it.

Robert Koch referred to the use of this assumption as the etiological standpoint.[16] It is the standpoint from which most medical research is carried out today — when it comes to disease, we think and work in terms of causes. Thus, when some new disease comes on the scene, we take for granted that the first step is to identify a causal factor in terms of which the disease can be characterized. This approach is now commonplace; we find almost unimaginable any other way of proceeding. And we have seen this approach used repeatedly with dramatic success over the last few decades: one must only think of infantile paralysis, AIDS, Legionnaires' Disease, and, more recently, SARS. Each has been and can be understood and controlled by assimilation to the etiological model.

The first cases of SARS are now believed to have emerged in mid-November 2002 in the Guangdong Province in China.[17] In February 2003, the disease, which was first characterized symptomatically as atypical pneumonia, was reported to the World Health Organization (WHO). Toward the end of February, a doctor from the Guangdong Province, who had treated patients now known to have had SARS, checked into a room on the ninth floor of a hotel in Hong Kong. By the time he arrived, he was displaying respiratory symptoms. Over the next few days, 12 other visitors and guests on the ninth floor of the hotel became ill. These victims, and other carriers, transported the disease further.

By the middle of March, the WHO knew that the world was threatened by a major new epidemic. By late March, various possible causal agents had been identified in the literature. Some evidence pointed to a paramyxovirus, but one writer observed that the "possible suspects" also included a parvovirus and a hantavirus.[18] By the end of March, just over one month after the first cases were reported to the WHO, researchers at the US Centers for Disease Control and Prevention (CDC) concluded that the causative agent was likely to be a new coronavirus.[19] CDC scientists had "cultured a coronavirus from tissue samples from two patients [and] also found it to occur specifically in lung and kidney tissues affected by the disease;" moreover, researchers found that "one patient started producing antibodies to the virus as the infection progressed."[20] By the middle of April, a consensus had emerged that the new coronavirus was the cause of SARS. In May, a research team announced having fulfilled R.J. Huebner's causal criteria for viruses[21] that were based on Koch's postulates.[22]

While the etiology of SARS is still not entirely clear, from my point of view, SARS represents just one more case in which a new disease has been successfully assimilated to the etiological standpoint — to the causal model that emerged in the middle of the nineteenth century and still dominates our thinking today. Research on SARS shows vividly how effective prophylaxis and (potentially) treatment and how orderly comprehension of disease phenomena become possible within the etiological standpoint.

Can all diseases be assimilated to the etiological standpoint? It isn't a fact about the world that some illnesses come packaged together with universal necessary causes; rather it is a fact about how we have learned to characterize diseases. When possible, we define diseases in terms of causes because there is great utility in doing so. But there may be diseases for which this is impossible either in principle or simply in fact.

Take an analogy from physics. Given a lump of purified uranium, it is impossible, *in principle*, to explain why one unstable atom decays at a certain time while surrounding, identical atoms do not. As currently understood, there is no sufficient cause for such an event; it simply happens. This seems to be a *metaphysical* issue, not an *epistemological* one; it stems from the way the world is, not from the weakness of our intellects. By a loose analogy, there could be individual disease episodes whose beginnings have no sufficient causes; they simply happen. Suppose there are such cases — some may even be sufficiently similar symptomatically that they can be grouped and labelled. Even so, it would obviously be false that all the members of such a group share the same sufficient cause; thus, an etiological definition and universal necessary causes would also be impossible. If this is how the world turns out to be, the very most one could hope for may be risk factors.

Alternatively, there could be disease episodes that do share sufficient causes, but causes whose identification requires more intellectual, financial, and/or temporal assets than we humans will ever have available. In short, there could be causes we are simply not smart enough to grasp.

As a species, we have spent more time and money on cancer research than on any other single scientific problem in our history. While we have learned a lot, we may be no closer to identifying sufficient causes in terms of which cancer (or even most specific classes of cancers) can be characterized than we were one hundred years ago. This could be because there simply are no such causes, or it could be because so far (and maybe forever) we are not smart enough to find them.

Through the last several decades, several disorders have emerged that seem also to defy characterizations that yield universal necessary causes: most psychological disorders seem to be this way as do obesity, depression, autism, attention deficit disorder, lupus, and a surprising variety of other problems. It may simply be impossible to account for these diseases following the usual causal model. It *may* be impossible, but of course we cannot be absolutely sure. Perhaps it will turn out that there is some kind of specific causal mechanism behind each such disorder; perhaps something different from anything we can currently imagine. Lacking a theory that tells us there are no causes (a sort of medical quantum theory), we cannot be sure that no causes will ever be found. Thus, even if there are illnesses without sufficient causes, it is not clear how we could ever come to know it, and in the absence of such knowledge, we could continue seeking non-existent causes for as long as we all shall live.

While the etiological standpoint has had enormous success, one cannot assume that every disease can be assimilated to this way of thinking. In time, it may not even prove to have been the best approach. So what does the future hold? Certainly, at this point, there is no clear alternative to approaching diseases causally. There is no going back to a system based predominantly on symptoms: having tasted the fruit of reliable control and of causal explanations, we are unlikely to be content with anything less whatever its virtues. One can imagine, just barely, a medical system in which risk factors replace universal necessary causes — this requires only a change, albeit a dramatic one, *within* the etiological framework. It would mean that control and explanation reduce to probabilities and thereby become much less reliable and much more difficult. Right now this is the best we can do for cancer and for the psychological disorders; perhaps this is the most we will ever achieve. But that would still be a medical system based on causes, and at this point it is virtually impossible to imagine how any future medical system could be organized except around some causal concepts or other.

But now we are beyond the limits to which philosophy can take us. Philosophy, like history, is inherently retrospective — it may help us understand the past, but it sheds little light on the future. Hegel put it this way: "When philosophy paints its gray in gray, then has a shape of life grown old.... The owl of Minerva spreads its wings only with the falling of the dusk."[23] Causal thinking in medicine may be on the brink of a revolution; but if so, it is a revolution to which neither historians nor philosophers are likely to contribute. Those of us on the outside can only wait and watch.

NOTES

[1]Wilhelm Friedrich Scanzoni, "[Review of] Skoda['s], Ueber die von Dr. Semmelweis entdeckte wahre Ursche der in der Wiener Gebäranstalt ungewönlich häufig vorkommenden Erkrankungen der Wöchnerinen," *Vierteljahrschrift für das praktische Heilkunde*, Literarische Anzeiger 26 (1845):25-33, see p. 32.

[2]A.F. Chomel, "Pneumonie," in *Dictionnaire de médecine*, 2nd edition, 30 vols., ed. Nicholas Philibert Adelon (Paris: Bechet, 1832–1846), Vol. XXV, pp. 165-66.

[3]James L. Bardsley, "Diabetes," in *Cyclopaedia of Practical Medicine*, American edition, 4 vols., ed. Robley Duglison (Philadelphia: Lea and Blanchard, 1845), Vol. I, p. 609.

[4]Gabriel Andral, "Hydrophobia," *Lancet* 1 (1832/33):806.

[5]K. Codell Carter, *The Rise of Causal Concepts of Disease* (Aldershot, UK: Ashgate Publishing Company, 2003).

[6]In this discussion, a *sufficient* cause is one in whose presence, other things being equal, a particular effect will always occur; a *necessary* cause is one in whose absence, other things being equal, a particular effect will not occur. A cause is *sufficient* for a certain effect if, given the cause, the effect always occurs; a cause is *necessary* for a certain effect if, given the effect, the cause always has occurred. For example, squishing a fly always leads to the death of the fly, so squishing is sufficient for killing a fly; moreover, if there is a fire, fuel has always been ignited, so fuel is necessary for fire. However, squishing is not necessary for the death of the fly because dead flies have not always been squished, and fuel is not sufficient for fire because wood may just rot away and never happen to be ignited.

[7]Jacob Henle, "Medicinische Wissenschaft und Empirie," *Zeitschrift für rationelle Medizin* 1 (1844):1-35.

[8]Danièle Ghesquier, "A Gallic Affair: The Case of the Missing Itch-Mite in French Medicine in the early 19th Century," *Medical History* 43 (1999):26-54.

[9]Philip Ricord, *Traité pratique des maladies vénériennes* (Paris: Just Rouvier et E. Le Bouvier, 1838).

[10]Agostino Bassi, *Del mal del segno, calcinaccio o moscardino*, ed. G.C. Ainsworth, trans. P.J. Yarrow (Ithaca, NY: Phytopathological Classics, Number 10, 1958).

[11]S.J. Zakon and T. Benedek, "David Gruby and the Centenary of Medical Mycology 1841–1941," *Bulletin of the History of Medicine* 16 (1944):155-68.

[12]K. Codell Carter, "Ignaz Semmelweis, Carl Mayrhofer, and the Rise of the Germ Theory," *Medical History* 29 (1985):353-74.

[13]Koch's Postulates are a set of criteria used to identify causes of diseases (originally bacterial diseases). In the 1880s, Robert Koch and his successors identified numerous non-equivalent sets. These sets usually required that the supposed cause can be identified in every examined case of the disease, that it can be isolated from diseased animals and (usually), after having been grown in inert media, can be used to

induce new cases of the disease when inoculated into healthy animals, and that its presence can explain disease phenomena.

[14]Eduard Lumpe, "Zur Theorie der Puerperalfieber," *Zeitschrift der k.k. Gesellschaft der Aerzte zu Wien* 6 (1850):392-98, see p. 392. The reference is to a trick, allegedly performed by Christopher Columbus and also by Filippo Brunelleschi, to make an egg stand on its small end; impossible for anyone until shown how: by tapping it to break a bit of the shell.

[15]Antoine Lavoisier, *Elements of Chemistry*, Great Books of the Western World, ed. Robert M. Hutchins (Chicago: Encyclopaedia Britannica), Vol. XXXXV, p. 1.

[16]Robert Koch, "Massnahmen gegen die Pest," in *Gesammelte Werke von Robert Koch*, ed. J. Schwalbe (Leipzig: George Thieme, 1912), p. 905.

[17]The following brief account of the history of SARS is based on (no author) "Communicable Disease Surveillance and Response: Severe Acute Respiratory Syndrome (SARS)" (Geneva: World Health Organization, 2003).

[18]M. Enserink, "Infectious Diseases: Scientists Chase Fast-Moving and Deadly Global Illness," *Science* 299 (21 March 2003):1822.

[19]H. Pearson, "Mystery Virus Slow to Yield its Identity as Patient Numbers Rise," *Nature* 422 (27 March 2004):1364.

[20]M. Enserink, "A Second Suspect in the Global Mystery Outbreaks," *Science* 299 (28 March 2003):1963.

[21]Robert J. Huebner, "The Virologist's Dilemma," *Annals of the New York Academy of Science* 67 (1957):430-38.

[22]Ron A.M. Foucher *et al.*, "Aetiology: Koch's Postulates Fulfilled for SARS Virus," *Nature* 423 (15 May 2003):240.

[23]G.W.F. Hegel, *Philosophy of Right*, Great Books of the Western World, ed. Robert M. Hutchins (Chicago: Encyclopaedia Britannica, 1952), Vol. XXXXVI, p. 7.

6

From Cholera to SARS: Communicable Disease-Control Procedures in Toronto, 1832 to 2003

Heather A. MacDougall

Introduction

In his recently released thriller *Pandemic*,[1] Dr. Daniel Kalla drew on his experience as the emergency room doctor who helped to contain Vancouver's only case of SARS to posit the use of disease as bio-terrorism and to highlight the need for more effective preparations to prevent and control such outbreaks. His hero, Professor Noah Haldane, an infectious disease specialist who works as a trouble-shooter for the World Health Organization (WHO), opens the story with the observation that SARS "has been good for us" because

> SARS put global infectious disease control measures to the test. And guess what? Not one country came up smelling like a rose. In fact, most stunk. Take Canada. Despite boasting one of the world's best health care systems, my colleagues in Toronto didn't react fast enough to the first case of SARS. And the city ended up paying dearly for it ... But at least now the world has been warned. We have the chance to fine-tune — in some cases revamp completely — our public health measures. In that sense, SARS was a good dry run for the real McCoy.[2]

But is this characterization of SARS' impact accurate or is it an example of artistic licence? Kalla has Haldane continue his lecture to medical students with a presentation on the 1918 flu pandemic — again to drive home the point that society is as unprepared for an international outbreak of influenza today as it was nearly 90 years ago, and, in fact, society may be more vulnerable because of the speed of air transportation.[3]

As Canadians discovered in March 2003, reality can be as frightening as fiction because it challenges a society's deeply held values and undermines facile assumptions about the superiority of scientific knowledge. When the SARS outbreak started, experts, health authorities, politicians, and the public all asked the following questions: How would a country that had not faced an epidemic disease of unknown origin and virulence for nearly half a century respond to the challenge of controlling the outbreak? Would citizens be willing to undergo traditional disease-control measures such as isolation and quarantine? Was the curative system prepared to cope with an influx of critically-ill patients? Who would serve as the official spokesperson? How could the public be kept informed but not frightened? Who would be responsible for paying the expenses of the sick, people in quarantine, and people whose jobs were adversely affected? And how would the three levels of government interact to protect citizen's health?

For Toronto Public Health, the arrival of SARS highlighted the never-ending challenge which local health departments face and have faced in controlling outbreaks. By examining the rise and evolution of methods for communicable disease control in Toronto during the nineteenth and twentieth centuries, we can see how epidemics shaped attitudes and behaviour,[4] contributed to the development of bacteriology and virology,[5] and gradually required governments at all levels to create administrative procedures that focused on both control and prevention.[6] From the fatalism that dominated lay and medical attitudes to cholera and typhus in the mid-nineteenth century to the belief that communicable disease had been "conquered" through adoption of the germ theory of disease causation and the discovery of vaccines to prevent diphtheria and polio, the work of local boards of health expanded not only to encompass four specific disease-control strategies — notification, isolation, quarantine, and terminal disinfection — but also to provide advice and guidance on the best measures to prevent the disease. All of these activities provoked both opposition and support and provided a demonstration of "fundamental patterns of social value and institutional practice."[7] But by the early twenty-first century, most of the long-established disease-control measures had disappeared because municipal health departments had ceased to placard houses for infectious diseases, closed their isolation hospitals, eliminated municipal diagnostic laboratories, and turned their attention to health promotion and be-haviour-modification programs between the 1960s and the 1990s.[8] And then SARS appeared. By comparing and contrasting the impact of epidemics of cholera, typhus, smallpox, and influenza on public attitudes to disease control and governmental responsibility, we will be able to assess the SARS outbreak in its historical context and determine the lessons that it had to teach politicians, bureau-crats, health authorities, infectious disease control experts, and citizens.

GOD'S SCOURGE OR MAN-MADE DISASTERS? EPIDEMIC DISEASE CONTROL, 1832–1900

Cholera

For early and mid-nineteenth-century cities and towns in British North America, the threat of epidemic outbreaks was an annual event because the arrival of immigrants often brought disease. Cholera epidemics in 1832, 1834, 1849, 1854, and 1866 were complemented by typhus in 1847 and smallpox in 1872–73, 1885, and 1888.[9] Cholera, in particular, was feared because it did not conform to prevailing medical theory, which postulated that miasmatic exhalations from rotting refuse caused atmospheric change, producing disease. Like SARS, cholera was a "shock" disease in 1832 and 1834 because it struck erratically and violently, produced horrifying symptoms, and did not respond to the heroic measures such as bleeding and the use of calomel, a purgative drug, recommended by regular medical men.[10] Since its initial victims were the poor, the dissolute, and the immigrants, the more affluent portion of soci-ety was prepared to view this as a divine scourge sent to remind society of its failings. But as subsequent epidemics demonstrated, cholera did not discrimi-nate and middle and upper classes perished as well. What impact did this disease have on local governments and their citizens?

In the town of York, the provincial capital of Upper Canada (shortly to become Toronto), citizens and the lieutenant-governor, General Sir John Colborne, were well aware that the immigration season of 1832 would bring cholera because Great Britain had experienced a devastating outbreak in 1831.[11] A war hero from the Battle of Waterloo, Colborne was a decisive leader who allocated £500 to combat the disease by creating medical boards throughout the colony. This money was to provide funds for the care of the sick and to prompt York, Kingston, Hamilton, and other centres to institute the sanitation measures that British experts regarded as the principal method of preventing the spread of disease.

In fact, the first line of defence was the new quarantine station established at Grosse Isle in the St. Lawrence River. Here, the incoming immigrants were to be inspected and isolated in the hospital facilities if visibly sick. Otherwise, they were sent to Quebec City, Montreal, and on to ports along the shores of the Great Lakes. With no knowledge that cholera is a water-borne bacteria, limited attention was paid to protecting food and water supplies, with the result that emigrant sheds became a feature of lakefront centres as their minimal hospital facilities were rapidly overwhelmed by disease victims. For York, the arrival of 30,000 to 40,000 immigrants in the summer of 1832 led to the creation of a medical board staffed by the town's 14 doctors and supported by the resolute efforts of lay and religious leaders who provided care for the sick. Prior to their arrival, the lieutenant-governor had ordered a day of "Public Fasting, Prayer and Humiliation" on Wednesday, 16 May 1832 to seek divine intervention to prevent the "great calamity" that was devastating other British colonies.[12] But for a portion of the more affluent inhabitants flight was the only answer. This spread the disease more widely and highlighted a common feature of epidemics: the contrast between those who stayed to fight the disease and those whose primary interest was self-preservation.

In addition to their curative role, the board also prepared regulations modelled on the British experience and demanded that citizens whitewash their premises, remove any human, animal, or vegetable waste, and use quicklime as a disinfectant.[13] Persuading the 5,505 inhabitants to follow these recommendations was as difficult as persuading the sick to enter the cholera hospital. The poor and immigrants feared being taken from their families because most early hospitals had reputations as death houses and York's was no exception. Indeed, rumours began to circulate that some of the sick were being buried alive and there was growing opposition to the requirement for prompt burial in lime-soaked winding sheets.[14] Conflict among the doctors also undercut the effectiveness of the board and it resigned in early August.[15] At the end of the epidemic in September, the official death count was 535 cases and 205 deaths, but both Bishop John Strachan and William Lyon Mackenzie, the radical reformer, stated that this underestimated total morbidity and mortality by half.[16]

What lessons had been learned? Clearly, the imposition of British-style regulations to prevent and control epidemics had not been an effective approach due to poor funding, indifferent public support, and variable understanding about the cause of the disease. As well, the roles of local and central authorities had not been clearly defined; with the result that York's board of health, like others, sought more money and expanded legal powers from the lieutenant-governor. But as the Legislative Assembly was not recalled during the epidemic, the chain of command issue was not dealt with until February 1833 when the Assembly passed *An Act to establish Boards of Health and to guard against the introduction of Malignant, Contagious and Infectious Diseases, in this Province*. This legislation permitted the creation of local boards of health during medical emergencies and represented the first formal attempt at state intervention in public health matters in Upper Canada.[17] Since this legislation lapsed within a year, the emerging towns and cities were left to develop their own approaches to disease control. When Toronto achieved municipal status in March 1834, the new city council with Mackenzie as its mayor passed a series of bylaws to create a framework for growth and development. Bylaw number 8 dealt with public health issues and was a direct response to the failure of 1832 disease-control efforts. The local business people who formed the council firmly believed in the miasmatic theory of disease causation, which viewed environmental problems as the cause of disease outbreaks; hence, a Local Board of Health was to be appointed annually to ensure that the city was properly scavenged in preparation for the arrival of potentially disease-ridden immigrants. If disease appeared, the Local Board of Health was to prepare buildings to serve the sick, set the rules for admission, hire medical and nursing staff, and provide food and other necessities at public expense. The opposition to hospitalization, which had occurred in 1832, was to be dealt with through fines and all doctors, innkeepers, hoteliers, and boarding-house keepers were required to report cases of disease to the authorities so that proper control measures could be implemented promptly.[18]

This bylaw was passed on 9 June 1834, but little action had been taken when the first cholera cases appeared at the end of July. Although the Local Board of Health was appointed, political factionalism between its Tory and Reform members and lack of money for sewers and scavenging rendered it ineffective, and once again Sir John Colborne provided emergency funds to ensure that the hospital opened. Between 1 and 15 August, 315 deaths were reported, and from 15 to 31 August there were 167 cholera death burials. As the epidemic came to an end in September, at least 500 people had perished and in contrast to 1832 there had been less effort made to inform the public about the situation and to encourage sanitary improvements.[19] Thus, Toronto's response to cholera in 1834 not only demonstrated the extent to which contemporary political frustrations, anxieties, and ideologies affected behaviour, but also demonstrated that epidemics do not always result in improved public health services.

The initial cholera epidemics aroused conflicting responses in Toronto and other colonial centres. Was the disease contagious or did it arise from environmental insanitation? How could citizens be persuaded to clean their homes and businesses as a preventive measure? Should towns and cities publish daily morbidity and mortality rates or did that just threaten their economic survival? Who should be sent to the temporary hospitals and should these be funded through local taxes, emigrant head taxes, or central expenditures? What role did the British government have in policing the flood of immigrants? All of these questions remained unanswered until the famine migration of the 1840s.

Typhus

The failure of the Irish potato crop in 1845 to 1850 led to mass starvation, mass exodus, and outbreaks of typhus and cholera in Ireland, Great Britain, and North America. The British North American colonies were particularly affected because they were the principal recipients of the pauper emigration since the American governments had passed legislation prohibiting ship owners from landing diseased passengers and as a result generally received only the well-to-do.[20]

As the magnitude of the 1847 famine migration became clear, Toronto's local board led by Alderman George Gurnett began to press the council for funds to set up a hospital. When this failed, the board negotiated with the trustees of the Toronto General Hospital to rent that facility and the patients were moved to another building while the hospital was prepared for sick immigrants. Over 90,000 immigrants, many of whom were sick, arrived at Grosse Isle between May and November 1847. The facilities there were quickly overwhelmed as were all the hospitals and emigrant sheds elsewhere along the St. Lawrence and the Great Lakes. The centrally-paid emigrant agents were under instructions to forward the immigrants to their ultimate destination as quickly as possible, but the physical debility of many of the newcomers not only made them vulnerable to typhus but also limited their ability to find work. Only grudgingly was the colonial government prepared to allow food and shelter for six days to help the immigrants adapt to the new land. But for hard-pressed municipalities in the Canadas, even this assistance was welcome.[21]

In Toronto, starting in mid-June, Gurnett met with his fellow Local Board of Health members daily at 10 in the morning to discuss the next steps in controlling the outbreak. After hiring Dr. George Grasett as both the city's medical health officer and the medical superintendent of the hospital, the board also decided to employ Constable John Townsend to inspect immigrants and their property as they arrived in the city and to prepare statistical reports. All of the city's papers printed Townsend's lists of cases, deaths, and convalescent cases, and several also provided summaries of the daily board meetings. Early in the outbreak the need for additional accommodation became clear, and eventually, 14 sheds were built. At the lakefront, two boilers for hot water were provided as well as fire wood and soap so that immigrants could clean themselves, their clothing, and their bedding. Since typhus is a rickettsial disease in which rats and body lice are vectors, cleaning the immigrants and their possessions was a useful preventive measure, but as the *British Colonist* noted, the newcomers could not be forced to carry out this action.[22]

A similar problem faced the Local Board of Health when it created "sanatory [sic] regulations" in late June. Torontonians were told that they were to report any cases of disease brought by immigrants and not to take any baggage or bedding into hotels or boarding houses unless they had been inspected by the town constables upon arrival. In spite of this clear-cut regulation, Constable Townsend and a colleague discovered many sick families in lodging houses, and like their predecessors in the 1830s, they encountered great resistance to hospitalization.[23] This was compounded as lay and medical caregivers succumbed; both Dr. Grasett and Toronto's Roman Catholic Bishop Michael Power died while many of the other medical staff along with George Gurnett contracted the disease but survived.[24]

From May to October, 29,613 immigrants arrived in Toronto: 3,300 were admitted to the General Hospital where 757 died, 1,993 were discharged, and 739 remained for further care.[25] For a city of 30,000 dealing with such a large number of sick and destitute newcomers challenged both the capacity for compassion and its economic stability. From the beginning, the mayor and city council had assumed that the central government would provide the funds to pay for the extra expenses that the outbreak caused. They did not know that the British government was telling the governor general, Lord Elgin, to keep expenses to a minimum and that many of his letters to the colonial secretary, Lord Grey, contained repeated arguments in favour of central funding. Eventually the mother country agreed to pay half the costs of the epidemic, but Elgin was told to assist the colonial assembly in designing legislation that would ensure that future outbreaks were handled and paid for by Canadians.[26]

In Toronto, both the Tory *British Colonist* and the Reform *Examiner* produced articles in which they castigated the British government for failing to inspect the immigrants prior to departure and for not ensuring that they had adequate food, water, and medical assistance during the voyage. The *Examiner* was so incensed by conditions on the "coffin-ships" that they were compared to the slave trade. Like their counterparts in Montreal and Quebec, both Toronto papers demanded changes to protect the public's health and to prevent British North America from being used as a dumping ground for the economic problems of the Irish and English landowners. Although the British government tightened immigration inspections and passed the 1848 *Public Health Act* which created a Central Board of Health just as the next cholera epidemic was about to arrive, most Canadians were focused on the election of the first purely Reform Party government in January 1848 and the revolutions that wracked Western Europe and Ireland that year. Only Bishop Strachan and Mayor George Gurnett took the possible threat of a cholera epidemic into consideration. In a pastoral letter of November 1848, the Bishop urged his parishioners to pray for divine support and pointed out that:

> Far greater attention is now paid to the cleanliness of our towns and cities — to the purifying of the atmosphere, to the better ventilation of the homes of the poor — to the encouragement of temperate habits — to the supply of warm clothing to the needy, and nourishing healthy food.... Moreover it has been shewn [sic] that cholera, in its first stage, is by no means unmanageable by simple remedies, and prompt recourse to medical assistance. One matter of great importance appears to be set at rest, namely, that cholera is not contagious, and that there is no risk in attending upon the sick and the dying. Now this is a most valuable discovery, for it will give confidence to the weak and timid to nurse their friends and neighbours, and the inmates of their families without fear or apprehension. During the last two visitations of the Pestilence, the poor were frequently much neglected. Pity was swallowed up by fear.... Now it is decided, by the best authorities, that there is far less danger in watching a Cholera patient than one in Typhus Fever.[27]

Mayor Gurnett warned his fellow citizens that with cholera reported in London and New York City in December, Toronto must begin to institute "precautionary and remedial measures" to prepare for the onslaught.[28]

Gurnett was re-elected as mayor in 1849 and on 5 March when the council committees were created, he was appointed to the Local Board of Health which was chaired by Alderman Joseph Workman, MD.[29] Workman had received his medical degree from McGill in 1835 after defending a thesis in which he argued that cholera was contagious. But it was his prowess as a businessman that had ensured his election to Toronto's council; he had served on the 1847 Local Board of Health and thus had experience with the challenges of controlling and preventing epidemic disease. In June, the Local Board of Health requested funds to construct a cholera hospital and was given £75 to do so. On a site in the western portion of the city, a wooden reception shed *cum* hospital was erected in spite of a flurry of petitions from local residents who opposed it. The inhabitants suggested constructing the building on the land adjacent to the Lunatic Asylum and when the shed was completed, much to Workman's chagrin, "a quarter of a dozen lofty magnates, residing in that region ... turned out one night and demolished our receiving house."[30] This mirrored a similar mob action in Quebec City and may well have taken its cue from the destruction of the Parliament Buildings in Montreal in April 1849. During the spring session of the Legislature, political conflict over the Rebellion Losses Bill had overshadowed the Baldwin-LaFontaine Ministry's passage of the 1849 *Act to Make Provision for the Preservation of the Public Health in Certain Emergencies*.[31] But the arrival of cholera in Kingston and its spread east and west along the St. Lawrence prompted the Governor-in-Council to bring the act into effect in early June through the creation of a Central Board of Health.

The purpose of the Canadian Central Board of Health was to provide advice and guidance through a set of regulations and bylaws that local boards were expected to administer. Made up of doctors and businessmen, the board reflected the mid-nineteenth-century view that medical expertise needed to be tempered by fiscal realism and conventional morality. Only the deserving poor were to receive assistance and all municipalities were expected to use their own taxes to pay for inspection and curative services. In Toronto, Workman resigned both his aldermanic seat and his Local Board of Health chairmanship after discovering that some of his council colleagues supported mob violence, leaving Gurnett and the rest of the board to contend with the epidemic.

The legislation provoked significant opposition in Toronto because the city was suffering from the economic downturn of 1847–48 and was strongly opposed to paying the costs for sick immigrants. Only after several public meetings had allowed opponents to vent their anger was a new board appointed once cases of cholera appeared. From July to September, 208 cases of cholera with 140 deaths occurred among immigrants while 565 Torontonians caught the disease and 329 died. In addition to demonstrating the fallacy that only immigrants would succumb, the outbreak marked the end of efforts to get full funding from senior levels of government.[32]

The cholera and typhus epidemics provided object lessons in the development of public policy. The announcement of impending disease provoked both panic and, in contrast, determination to care for the sick and prevent the spread of the illness. With local papers reporting medical and scientific theories of disease causation and prevention, printing the regulations provided by senior governments, commenting favourably or critically on municipal efforts, and advertising patent medicines and home remedies, citizens who were literate could draw their own conclusions about the danger of remaining and their chances of survival if they undertook charitable activity. In such a strongly Christian community, religious beliefs dictated acceptance of God's will and encouraged compassion for the sick and destitute. For the immigrants who were viewed as the source of disease, epidemics meant the death of loved ones, the denial of traditional burial practices, and a negative reaction from some members of the host society. Given the episodic nature of the disease outbreaks and the limited knowledge of disease causation, Toronto's citizens, the newcomers, and the local boards of health all responded to each epidemic with a mixture of hope and fear. But the fatalism that guided many was gradually being replaced with an expectation that medical science would uncover the cause of disease and then develop effective preventive measures.

Throughout this period, civic politicians shared the beliefs of their constituents but were also deeply concerned about central interference unless it was accompanied by funding. The drive to achieve responsible government for the United Canadas was paralleled by local determination to remain free to respond to local needs and concerns, not simply to be creatures of the provincial government. For Toronto, this meant controlling the costs of epidemics through careful expenditure on curative and preventive services and sustained efforts to regain trade and tourism after each outbreak was over.[33] Only with the city's rapid expansion at the end of the century would it also encompass permanent staff and measures to protect public health.

CONTROLLING COMMUNICABLE DISEASE: BUREAUCRACY AND BACTERIOLOGY

In spite of further cholera epidemics in 1854 and 1866, Canadian politicians did not see controlling communicable disease as a national activity except for maintaining quarantine stations and caring for sick mariners. Instead, health, education, and municipal institutions were left to the provinces who formed the new Canadian federation. In Ontario, the first post-Confederation public health act in 1873 was permissive legislation which quickly failed to meet the challenge of urban-industrial growth. A Sanitary Commission established in 1878 reported to the Mowat government and, like its British counterparts, argued vehemently that permanent local boards with medical health officers and sanitary inspectors were an essential component of urban life if the state wished to ensure the health of its citizens and continuing productivity. In 1882, the Provincial Board of Health was created to provide advice to local boards regarding communicable disease-control procedures and standards for environmental sanitation. During the same period, the Canadian Medical Association had been pressing the federal government to collect mortality statistics and in 1883 the Macdonald administration introduced a conditional grant for this purpose. Cities with populations of 10,000 to 25,000 were eligible for funding if they had a medical health officer who provided the mortality returns. Since Toronto had a population of roughly 86,000 and was the second largest city in the Dominion, the city council decided to appoint a full-time medical health officer, both to qualify for the federal grant and to deal with the rising morbidity and mortality that occurred as the city grew. Dr. William Canniff, the first full-time medical officer of health appointed in March 1883 was a prominent British-trained surgeon, medical educator, and Canadian nationalist, who strongly believed in contingent-contagionism, and therefore focused his attention on improving Toronto's sanitation.[34]

Smallpox

In 1885 and again in 1888, Canniff had to battle smallpox. In contrast to the cholera and typhus epidemics, the smallpox outbreaks did not erupt as a result of immigration. Instead, the disease was endemic, but since it increased and decreased in virulence, the milder form was often mistaken for chickenpox or measles. Canniff's medical colleagues, however, were more than willing to report cases of this dangerous disease to his office so that he and his slowly growing staff of inspectors could take control. The 1885 outbreak enabled the Medical Health Department to develop its standard procedures for disease control by adapting portions of the model health bylaw which had been appended to the 1884 *Provincial Public Health Act*. Prompt notification; in-house inspection to confirm the disease; vaccination of family, friends, and co-workers; isolation of the disease victim; quarantine of close contacts; fumigation of the premises; and eventually opening a city smallpox hospital with a sentry to protect the sick from irate residents became Toronto's *modus operandi*. The whole system was predicated on persuading the sick and their families to accept supervision by the health department. This strategy did not suffice for the Provincial Board of Health which had taken a much more activist stance to protect Ontario. The board had sent staff to Montreal to inspect goods being shipped west and to examine train passengers for proof of recent vaccinations. The extent of the Quebec outbreak with more than 9,000 deaths and nearly 19,000 cases led the Provincial Board of Health to advocate mass vaccination. Toronto's medical officer of health and its local board resisted because the city had only 28 cases of the disease with three deaths and because voluntary vaccination was being carried on successfully.[35]

When the disease reappeared in 1888, the medical officer of health and his staff re-implemented their recently-developed procedures, but this time they faced a vocal anti-vaccination campaign led by Dr. Alexander M. Ross who argued that vaccination was only applied to poor working men and women and their children, not to the "better classes." His views had little impact because citizens in the affected areas flocked to the public vaccination stations in such numbers that the health department ran out of lymph. Early in October new cases of the disease appeared just as fresh supplies of vaccine arrived and the epidemic was controlled by November. But like the 1885 outbreak, this too was productive of discord between the province and the capital city. The Provincial Board of Health secretary, Dr. Peter H. Bryce, was intent on demonstrating the effectiveness of preventive measures and therefore objected to lack of compulsory vaccination and placarding of infected homes and businesses in Toronto. Canniff and the Local Board of Health were concerned about the city's reputation, its economy, and the privacy of disease victims, their families and their doctors.[36] Toronto's medical officer of health argued:

> As to the advisability of reporting all cases of infectious disease to the Provincial Board of Health, Dr. Canniff considers it no part of the duty of that body

to officiously interfere with local boards unless they are failing in their duty. It is discretionary with local boards ... to make known or otherwise of cases of infectious disease, but in Toronto it has been the practice to give the public all the facts wherever any benefit could possibly accrue.[37]

At the same time that Canniff and his staff were pioneering their disease-control techniques, medical researchers were uncovering the bacterial causes of tuberculosis, cholera, diphtheria, gonorrhea, and other communicable diseases.[38] For Canniff's successors, integrating this new knowledge into communicable disease-control procedures resulted in the construction of a permanent Isolation Hospital in 1892–93, the creation of a municipal bacteriological laboratory in 1894, and the use of toxin-anti-toxin treatment for diphtheria.[39] As the provincial capital, Toronto became the centre of medical education and a focal point for advances in public health through the creation of the Connaught Laboratories in 1914 and the appointment of Charles Hastings as the medical officer of health in 1910. Hastings was a proponent of the "new public health" with its focus on health education and disease prevention rather than disease control and sanitation. Under his dynamic direction, Toronto's health department expanded to include a corps of public health nurses, municipal housekeepers, more laboratory staff and statisticians, as well as public health inspectors.[40]

Not only did he encourage professional qualifications for his staff, but Hastings also used the media and his public addresses to educate citizens, politicians, and colleagues about their responsibilities for ensuring their own and their families' healths. The monthly *Health Bulletin* which the department distributed to voluntary groups, school teachers, and parents regularly contained brief articles highlighting the location of well-baby and tuberculosis clinics along with reminders to parents and practitioners not to ignore sore throats in children because it was vital to administer the toxin-anti-toxin treatment as soon as possible. Using the reportable diseases listed in the revised provincial *Public Health Act* of 1912 as a guide, the health department's Division of Communicable Disease Control maintained vigilant oversight of Toronto's health during the First World War.

Influenza

In 1918–19, however, the Department of Public Health faced a new enemy — influenza. When the epidemic began in late September, Hastings found himself in the same position as his predecessors because the cause of the disease was unknown, it was not reportable, and had apparently acquired increased virulence which made its rapid spread particularly lethal among young adults rather than its usual victims. Although the standard disease-control procedures were attempted, the city's hospitals quickly filled to capacity and health-care personnel fell victim to the disease.[41] The health department immediately modified its regular duties and focused on combating the outbreak. The public health nurses continued their home visits and attempted to provide as much nursing care as possible while inspectors from the various divisions were put in charge of providing fuel and other necessities to stricken families on a 24-hour basis.[42]

The medical officer of health persuaded the Local Board of Health to support his restrictions on public gatherings and to fund the creation of emergency hospital facilities because the health department was dealing with more of the sick than existing hospitals. The Academy of Medicine approved the medical officer of health's efforts and recommended delaying elective surgery until the epidemic was over, while the University of Toronto School of Dentistry closed its public clinic for the duration and the Medical Faculty asked its senior students to volunteer to assist local doctors or to work in Department of Public Health (DPH) hospitals.[43]

As the number of cases increased, the war effort was slowed since munitions production and train transport were affected. By 23 October, 54 of 319 DPH staff were ill, including 22 nurses, and four doctors and volunteers were desperately needed.[44] Prior to the war, the Department of Public Health had assisted with the formation of the Neighbourhood Worker's Association and this group in conjunction with the IODE, Toronto Women's Liberal Association, and women's church groups worked to staff soup kitchens, make pneumonia jackets, collect bedding and clothing, and distribute them to the sick. But who was going to pay for these activities? As the extent of the epidemic became clear, the Board of Trade supported the creation of an Influenza Fund to provide money to assist poverty-stricken families and asked the Federation of Community Services to act as the distribution agent.[45] By the end of the epidemic, health department staff had made 17,108 visits to stricken households and records indicate that 1,750 Torontonians had died.[46] Since there were probably in excess of 150,000 cases among the nearly 490,000 people living in the city, Hastings may well have been correct when he claimed that Toronto "passed through the influenza epidemic in one week less, and with a lower mortality than any other city of equal size."[47]

But as the gallant work of his staff, the hospital personnel, and the numerous volunteers had demonstrated, controlling the outbreak posed the same types of challenges as Torontonians had experienced in the nineteenth century. However, seeking to apply their bacteriological expertise, scientists in Western Europe and North America had attempted to develop a preventive or prophylactic vaccine, using strains of bacilli from flu victims.[48] But although the provincial public health laboratories, Connaught Laboratories, and the Toronto General Hospital laboratory all produced batches of vaccine based on American strains plus those derived from soldiers in Toronto's Base Hospital, none of these proved particularly effective. As the president of the American Public Health Association, Hastings was kept abreast of developments in the United States as well as in Canada, and as he indicated to the Toronto *Globe,* vaccines against flu were still at the experimental stage, so more traditional methods had to be used.[49] Indeed, British and Canadian medical officers noted prophylactic vaccination did little and suggested that the micro-organism that caused influenza was likely a filterable virus rather than Pfeiffer's bacillus.[50] Although they were proven correct in 1933, flu continues to be a constant concern for municipal health departments, which must remain alert to its potential transformation from nuisance disease to pandemic threat.

Diphtheria and Polio

In spite of the failure of medical science to prevent or control the great influenza pandemic, the twentieth century witnessed public acceptance of the "germ" theory and, at least in the developed world, the eradication and control of childhood killers such as diphtheria and poliomyelitis. Local health departments played a prominent role in these achievements because they worked with the press, non-governmental organizations such as the Health League of Canada, religious leaders, and radio stations to publicize the benefits of immunization programs. Toronto led the country in the development of annual Toxoid Weeks which emphasized the importance of preventing diphtheria in babies, preschoolers, and school-age children. By 1940 the city was unique because it had no cases and no deaths from the disease.[51]

But as Dr. Gordon Jackson, the medical officer of health from 1929 to 1951, ruefully noted, as soon as one scourge was controlled another appeared. During the 1930s, 1940s, and early 1950s, outbreaks of polio caused great fear and concern for parents. For local health departments, the disease posed a challenge since there was little that could apparently be done to prevent it and thus attention focused on controlling the spread. In 1937, Toronto experienced a devastating epidemic with 768 cases and 40 deaths. The city used the outbreak to conduct a clinical trial of preventive nasal spray, but this prophylactic failed to limit the spread of the disease. The health department also did yeoman work with local agencies and organizations such as the Kinsmen and Rotary Clubs to ensure that all victims of the disease received assistance, but press reports focused on apparent conflicts between the Board of Health and the Board of Education about opening the city's schools, whether the Board of Health had the right to prohibit Children's Day at the Canadian National Exhibition, and whether the public should be provided with full information about the extent of the epidemic. In the interests of the city's economic situation, the medical officer of health did not ban Children's Day, but did encourage parents to keep their children away from public venues. He supported the decision to keep the city's schools closed until the epidemic had run its course and then had all the public health nurses, aided by retired and married colleagues, provide inspection when the schools opened. Their efforts uncovered several cases of the disease, but also served to assure parents that the epidemic was over.[52] The development of the Salk vaccine provided the first effective preventive measure and Toronto's health department launched its mass immunization campaign among school children in 1955. The advent of the Sabin oral vaccine led to a Metro Toronto-wide effort by all the local health departments to get children and adults to swallow the new preventive.[53]

From Control to Prevention

The very success of these immunization campaigns and the declining morbidity rates from communicable diseases led to public complaisance and also prompted public health officials to rethink their priorities. By the early 1950s, Toronto no longer used placards to identify homes in which communicable disease was present, nor did it insist on fumigation. The city's Isolation Hospital was transformed into the Riverdale Chronic Care facility in 1957; that year as well, the city closed its bacteriological laboratory since provincial facilities were well able to conduct the tests as required. During the 1970s and 1980s, poverty and the diseases of affluence, as well as the needs of immigrants and the elderly, became the focal point of local health endeavours. During these decades, however, the arrival of immigrants and refugees with active cases of giardiasis, tuberculosis, and occasionally polio served to remind public health staff that the war against disease was never-ending.[54] In 1984 the new provincial *Health Protection and Promotion Act* reiterated the role that local departments and health units were expected to play in controlling communicable disease but also outlined an expanded set of mandatory programs which required extensive spending and the hiring of additional staff.

For Toronto, this legislation and the subsequent provincial cuts to preventive services funding made it challenging to deal with the appearance of HIV/AIDS in the 1980s. Focusing on health education rather than curative activities meant developing new strategies to disseminate information, finding allies within the affected communities, and hiring non-traditional staff to take the message to high-risk groups while at the same time dealing with the prejudice and fear manifested by many citizens.[55] In some respects, the AIDS pandemic illustrated both how far Toronto had come from the small nineteenth-century city with its *ad hoc* reaction to cholera and yet in others, how little had changed in terms of attitudes toward people who suffered from the disease.[56] But in contrast to the past, activist groups emerged to battle for attention, funding, and the right to participate in treatment decisions. By 1990 there was a national AIDS program and local health departments were now key partners in the battle against the disease.[57]

But were the lines of communication open? Was Toronto prepared for a major disease outbreak? In Canada, the HIV/AIDS epidemic unfolded against a backdrop of significant policy change in the health-care sector. During the Mulroney administration, the federal government imposed spending constraints on its portion of the social envelope; their Liberal successors continued this policy until 2000. At the provincial level, the Harris regime from 1995–2000 not only cut social funding but also unilaterally amalgamated Toronto and the five surrounding municipalities in 1997. Toronto Public Health thus was adapting to the unification of six unique health departments and facing sustained funding cuts on the eve of the millennium.[58] Although the terrorist attack of 11 September 2001 and the subsequent fears of smallpox and anthrax bio-terrorism started to compel the federal or provincial authorities to plan for a national disaster or the threat of a pandemic, little attention was paid to local public health activities. In 2002, influenza caused a rash of deaths in Ontario. Many of these were blamed on over-crowded emergency rooms and lack of medical and nursing staff, resulting from lack of funding. In response, the province began to prepare a flu pandemic plan and copied the Alberta strategy of providing free flu shots to citizens. But in February 2003 when SARS arrived in Toronto, neither of the senior levels had a clear or coherent plan for controlling and eradicating the disease in place.

SARS

As the Naylor, Walker and Campbell reports indicate, the SARS outbreak illustrated many weaknesses in the Canadian approach to disease containment.[59] But all agree that the work of Toronto Public Health was exemplary. Lacking basic disease reporting technology, limited by privacy legislation, and hamstrung by conflict between the federal and provincial authorities, Toronto Public Health staff and the city's medical officer of health, Dr. Sheela Basrur, focused their attention on calming public concern, tracking cases and contacts, persuading citizens to undertake voluntary quarantine and in-home isolation, and providing expert advice through hotlines and Internet links. Roughly 700 of the 1,800 staff of the department served as part of the team dealing with the outbreak. When the hotline opened, the daily volume of calls demonstrated the range of fears and concerns that the city's 1.4 million inhabitants expressed. Preparing print and Internet information sheets required careful attention since all material was translated into 14 different languages and cultural sensitivities had to be observed.[60] And most challenging of all, the medical officer of health had to appear at the daily press briefing in company with infectious disease experts from city hospitals, the province's chief medical officer and the chief of emergency measures, all of whom represented specific interests.[61] The visible tension between the provincial experts intensified as criticism of the province's efforts appeared in the media and federal experts were heard bemoaning their lack of knowledge. The result was the WHO imposition of a travel ban on the city even though most inhabitants were continuing with their lives and relying on the calm reassurances of the city's medical officer of health that the situation was under control.[62] By the time the second phase of the epidemic was over, Toronto had experienced 224 cases and 44 deaths from SARS. Nearly 30,000 people had been quarantined, but only 27 legal orders had been required to ensure compliance.

But like its nineteenth-century counterparts, the SARS outbreak had highlighted the weaknesses in Toronto and Canada's disease-control apparatus. Who was in charge? Who should be providing information to the various levels of government and international agencies? Who should coordinate quarantine support measures, Toronto Public Health or voluntary groups? To whom should the public turn for information on disease prevention? Who should be responsible for dealing with the economic costs and consequences of disease outbreaks? In the wake of the SARS crisis, clearer lines of command have been created. The federal government has established the Canadian Public Health Agency to coordinate national disease control and prevention strategies and to provide a point of contact with international bodies such as the WHO.[63] The McGuinty government has begun to implement some of the recommendations of the Walker and Campbell reports, starting with the creation of a provincial disaster relief team and the appointment of Dr. Basrur as the province's chief medical officer. Her mandate has been expanded to include control of emergency situations.[64] But what about the city's health department? No one who lived through the experience is likely to forget the anxiety and tension of the period from March to August 2003, especially since new cases seemed to appear on Fridays, thus requiring extensive overtime on weekends. But the camaraderie produced by facing and defeating such a foe cannot mask the psychological pain which Toronto Public Health and hospital staff faced when friends, neighbours, and even some family members regarded them as pariahs because they had dealt with or cared for SARS patients.[65]

CONCLUSION

For nearly two centuries, Toronto has faced repeated outbreaks of contagious disease and as this overview suggests, controlling and preventing cholera, typhus, smallpox, diphtheria, polio, HIV/AIDS, and SARS reflected the values of the society and its beliefs about disease causation. During the early nineteenth century, a firm belief that disease was imported prompted an episodic response until Toronto was large enough to experience rising morbidity and mortality rates that were associated with urban-industrial growth. The cholera and typhus epidemics revealed both the heroism and self-interest of citizens as the devout ministered to the sick and the fearful fled. Similar reactions continued in the twentieth century, but increasing faith in both medical expertise to reveal the cause and clinical course of communicable diseases, along with the ability of local authorities to provide sustained control and prevention measures, meant greater public support for specific measures such as in-home quarantine, isolation in the city's Isolation Hospital, and prompt reporting by the city's doctors. Although the senior levels of government provided advice and guidance, carrying out actions designed to protect the city's health and maintain its economy were the responsibility of the health department. Dynamic leadership by the city's medical health officers during smallpox, diphtheria, and polio crises created a tradition within the department that ensured that its staff and their fellow citizens responded effectively to epidemic outbreaks until the 1960s. But the disappearance of these killers and the shift from health education to health promotion meant that communicable disease control units were downgraded and staff reassigned to new duties. For Toronto, the continuing arrival of immigrants and refugees with active cases of tuberculosis and its resurgence in the homeless, Aboriginals, and individuals with compromised immune systems meant controlling and preventing communicable disease remained an ongoing responsibility. But such apparently routine activity was little preparation for SARS.

As Kalla argues, the SARS outbreak was indeed a wake-up call. The outbreak revealed how completely the disease-fighting apparatus and methods that had been built up through experience with epidemics and the great flu pandemic had been dismantled by cost constraints and the belief that medical science could protect society from disease. In an uncomfortable echo of the anti-Irish sentiment in the 1840s, the origins of SARS in China led to boycotts of Chinese businesses and prompted calls for more stringent immigration control by the federal authorities. But the most challenging aspect of the SARS outbreak was the lack of cooperation and coordination between federal, provincial, and local authorities. This is clearly not a new problem since similar difficulties have always occurred when governments are challenged by disease threats. But in an age of instantaneous communication through the Internet, cellphones and CNN, any lack of unanimity was immediately evident, and conflicts over the clinical course of the disease, the amount of time required in quarantine, and many other aspects of the disease-control effort were broadcast with little attention to their potential impact on the mental health and stability of city in which the disease was unfolding. As this historical analysis has demonstrated, creating and maintaining a flexible, culturally-sensitive, and efficient disease-control and prevention program requires cooperation and coordination by all levels of government in order to ensure that local health departments/ units can meet the challenges of the future. As the front line in the never-ending battle against communicable disease, they must have the resources and legal power to protect the community's health.

NOTES

[1] Daniel Kalla, *Pandemic: A Novel* (New York: A Tom Doherty Associates Book, 2005).

[2] Ibid., p. 10.

[3] Ibid., pp. 11-12. The rest of the novel provides a mixture of derring-do as the intrepid hero travels the world trying to find the source of a deadly disease that erupts in various key centres and very detailed information about how infectious disease organisms mutate and colonize the human body.

[4] See Charles E. Rosenberg, "Explaining Epidemics" and "What is an Epidemic? AIDS in Historical Perspective" in *Explaining Epidemics and Other Studies in the History of Medicine*, ed. Charles E. Rosenberg (New York: Cambridge University Press, 1992), pp. 293-304 and 278-92; Nancy Tomes, "Epidemic Entertainments: Disease and Popular Culture in Early-Twentieth-Century America," *American Literary History* 14 (Winter 2002):625-52; Margaret Humphreys, "No Safe Place: Disease and Panic in American History," *American Literary History* 14 (Winter 2002):845-57; and Martin S. Pernick, "Contagion and Culture," *American Literary History* 14 (Winter 2002):858-65.

[5] George Rosen, *A History of Public Health,* expanded edition (Baltimore and London: Johns Hopkins University Press, 1993); Paul A. Bator with A.J. Rhodes, *Within Reach of Everyone: A History of the University of Toronto School of Hygiene and the Connaught Laboratories,* Vol. 1, 1927–1955 (Ottawa: Canadian Public Health Association, 1990); Peter Radetsky, *Invisible Invaders: The Story of the Emerging Age of Viruses* (Boston: Little, Brown and Company, 1991).

[6] For the Canadian experience, see R.D. Defries, ed., *The Development of Public Health in Canada*, 1st edition (Toronto: Canadian Public Health Association, 1940); R.D. Defries, ed., *The Federal and Provincial Health Services in Canada* (Toronto: Canadian Public Health Association, 1959, 1962).

[7] Rosenberg, "What is an Epidemic? AIDS in Historical Perspective," p. 279.

[8] Heather MacDougall, *Activists and Advocates: Toronto's Health Department, 1883–1983* (Toronto: Dundurn Press, 1990); see also Benoît Gaumer, Georges Desrosiers and Othmar Keel, *Histoire du Service de santé de la ville de Montréal, 1865–1975* (Quebec: Les Presses de l'Université Laval, 2002); Maureen Riddell, *History of the Edmonton Local Board of Health, 1871–1980* (Edmonton, 1980).

[9] For cholera history, see Geoffrey Bilson, *A Darkened House: Cholera in Nineteenth-Century Canada* (Toronto: University of Toronto Press, 1980); and Charles Godfrey, *The Cholera Epidemics in Upper Canada* (Montreal: Seecombe House, 1968). For Toronto's experience in dealing with all these diseases, see Heather MacDougall, "'Health is Wealth': The Development of Public Health Activity in Toronto, 1832–1890." Unpublished doctoral dissertation. University of Toronto, 1981.

[10] As Geoffrey Bilson states: "The disease [cholera] is caused by a micro-organism which enters the body through the mouth. It can multiply without producing

symptoms, and can cause minor disturbances, or severe illness which can kill more than one-half of those affected ... It causes vomiting and massive purging ... In its course it produces a number of symptoms including spasms and cramps, a sunken face, blue colour, husky voice, and further consequences, including kidney failure, as the bodily processes collapse" (*A Darkened House*, p. 5). He also notes that early and mid-nineteenth century doctors' usual treatments were unavailing against the massive dehydration and loss of electrolytes which we treat with saline solution (ibid., pp. 143-65).

[11]See R.J. Morris, *Cholera 1832: The Social Response to an Epidemic* (London: Croom Helm, 1976); Margaret Pelling, *Cholera, Fever and English Medicine, 1825–1865* (London: Oxford University Press, 1978); and Dorothy Porter, *Health, Civilization and the State: A History of Public Health from Ancient to Modern Times* (London and New York: Routledge, 1999).

[12]Proclamation, *Upper Canada Gazette*, 26 April 1832; J.J. Heagerty, *Four Centuries of Medical History in Canada* (Toronto: Macmillan, 1928), Vol. 1, pp. 184-85.

[13]Bilson, *A Darkened House*, pp. 56-57; York Board of Health *Minutes,* 21, 22, 23, 24, 26, 29 June, 7, 17, 28 July 1832.

[14]Bilson, *A Darkened House*, pp. 58-59; Godfrey, *The Cholera Epidemics*, p. 25.

[15]Edith Firth, ed., *The Town of York, 1815–1834: A Further Collection of Documents of Early Toronto* (Toronto: The Champlain Society for the Government of Ontario/University of Toronto Press, 1966), pp. 245-52.

[16] Ibid., p. 253; *Colonial Advocate*, 9 August 1832.

[17]K.F. Brandon, "Public Health in Upper Canada," in *The Development of Public Health in Canada*, ed. Defries, pp. 61-66.

[18]MacDougall, "Health is Wealth," pp. 35-40.

[19]Bilson, *A Darkened House*, pp. 85-89; MacDougall, "Health is Wealth," pp. 40-42.

[20]Joseph Robins, *The Miasma: Epidemic and Panic in Nineteenth Century Ireland* (Dublin: Institute of Public Administration, 1995), pp. 153-54.

[21]A.G. Doughty, ed., *The Elgin-Grey Papers, 1846–1852,* Vol. 1 (Ottawa, 1937), pp. 58-64.

[22]*British Colonist*, 23 July 1847.

[23]*British Colonist*, 24 August 1847.

[24]For discussion on Dr. Grasett, see *Patriot*, 20 July 1847 and *British Colonist,* 20 July 1847; on 24 August 1847, the *Colonist* reported that three of the five Roman Catholic priests were sick and that Bishop Power was now doing all the Cathedral services and "constant visiting at the Hospital sheds." He died on 1 October 1847. See his entry in the *Dictionary of Canadian Biography* Vol. VII (Toronto: University of Toronto Press, 1988) or online at www.biographi.ca.

[25]*British Colonist*, 2 November 1847.

[26]Doughty, *Elgin-Grey Papers,* Vol. 1, pp. 69-103.

[27]John, Lord Bishop of Toronto, *Pastoral Letter, to the Clergy and Laity of the Diocese of Toronto on the Subject of The Cholera* (Toronto: Printed at the Diocesan Press, 1848) CIHM item 89833, pp. 11-12.

[28]*British Colonist*, 8 December 1848.

[29]*Dictionary of Canadian Biography*, Vol. XII, 1891–1900 (Toronto: University of Toronto Press, 1990).

[30]Joseph Workman, "Reminiscences of Asiatic Cholera in Canada," *Canada Lancet* 16 (1883/84):37.

[31]An act to make provision for the preservation of the Public Health in certain emergencies, 12 Victoria, Chapter 8, 25th April 1849, 2nd-3rd Parliament, Province of Canada Statutes, Laws etc. 1847–1848/49, Microfiche CA2 WX Reel 2.

[32]MacDougall, "Health is Wealth," pp. 65-71.

[33]In 1847, for example, the *British Colonist* had a brief news item, "The Health of the City," on 24 August in which it not only argued that Toronto had done a better job of dealing with the epidemic than Montreal and Kingston but that the Local Board of Health was justified in printing the daily returns of cases and deaths because such information would assure American visitors that "the city is in its usual healthy condition, and that sickness among its inhabitants has not been greater in this than in former years" and hence that "Toronto has all the charms she ever had and more, both for the invalid, and the pleasure seeker."

[34]Heather MacDougall, "Public Health in Toronto's Municipal Politics: The Canniff Years, 1883–1890," *Bulletin of the History of Medicine* 55, no. 2 (Summer 1981):186-202.

[35]MacDougall, "Health is Wealth," pp. 222-46.

[36]Ibid., pp. 247-63.

[37]*Toronto News*, 3 October 1888.

[38]See Rosen, *A History of Public Health,* pp. 270-319.

[39]MacDougall, *Activists and Advocates*, pp. 22-26, 138.

[40]MacDougall, *Activists and Advocates*, pp. 26-31, 51-69.

[41]*The Globe*, Thursday, 10 October 1918, p. 8 reported that 100 hospital nurses were sick.

[42]"Can Keep Down the Mortality," *The Globe*, Friday, 11 October 1918, p. 6.

[43]"Doctors Strive Hard to Kill Influenza Epidemic," *The Globe*, Saturday, 12 October 1918, p. 8; "31 Deaths in Toronto Ascribed to Influenza," *The Globe*, Thursday, 17 October 1918, p. 6.

[44]Eileen Pettigrew, *The Silent Enemy: Canada and the Deadly Flu, 1918* (Saskatoon: Western Producer Prairie Books, 1983), p. 53.

[45]"Want Follows 'Flu' Ravages," *The Globe*, Thursday, 31 October 1918, p. 10.

[46]Marion Royce, *Eunice Dyke: Health Care Pioneer* (Toronto: Dundurn Press, 1983), pp. 69-70. The *Canadian Journal of Medicine and Surgery* 45 (July 1919):212 states that Toronto suffered 1,408 deaths from influenza and 1,307 from pneumonia for a total of 2,715, which was 1,980 in excess of the normal October death rate of 735.

[47]"Toronto Has Best Record," *The Globe*, Friday, 15 November 1918, p. 9.

[48]Eugenia Tognotti, "Scientific Triumphalism and Learning from Facts: Bacteriology and the 'Spanish Flu' Challenge of 1918," *Social History of Medicine* 16, no. 1 (2003):97-110.

[49]"City Death Rate Falls Rapidly," *The Globe*, Wednesday, 30 October 1918, p. 9. For similar efforts in another Canadian city, see Esyllt Jones, "Co-operation in All Human Endeavour: Quarantine and Immigrant Disease Vectors in the 1918–1919 Influenza Pandemic in Winnipeg," *Canadian Bulletin of Medical History/Bulletin canadien d'histoire de la médecine* 22, no. 1 (2005):57-82.

[50]H.G. Gibson, F.B. Bowman and J.L. Connor, "A Filterable Virus as the Cause of the Early Stage of the Present Epidemic of Influenza," *British Medical Journal* (14 December 1918):645.

[51]Sidney M. Katz, "A City Without Diphtheria," *Health* 8(March 1941):17; MacDougall, *Activists and Advocates*, pp. 140-44.

[52]MacDougall, *Activists and Advocates*, pp. 148-52.

[53]Ibid., pp. 152-58.

[54]Ibid., pp. 196-98, 201-04, 207-10, 220-31.

[55]"Toronto's Grassroots Approach," *Health Promotion,* Summer 1990, pp. 27, 31.

[56]The *Annual Statements* published by Toronto's health department between 1983 and 1997 made it clear that HIV/AIDS was a significant issue. Minutes of Local Board of Health meetings for the same period contain numerous references to reports from the medical officer of health on issues such as negative stereotyping of Haitians as AIDS carriers, the role ACT (The AIDS Committee of Toronto) as a public educator and agitator with senior levels of government, and the legal status of the Local Board of Health and DPH in terms of operating The Works, a needle exchange program intended to limit the spread of the disease.

[57]"National AIDS Strategy and Federal Action Plan," *Health Promotion*, Summer 1990, pp. 11-13; see "Around the Regions," *Health Promotion*, Summer 1990, pp. 25-31 for information about other Canadian provinces and cities.

[58]David McKeown, *Public Health: Challenges in a Time of Transformation, Toronto Public Health 1996 Annual Statement* (Toronto, 1997); see also Toronto Public Health, *Public Health Budget Fact Sheet*, 10 March 1998.

[59]National Advisory Committee on SARS and Public Health, D. Naylor, *Learning from SARS: Renewal of Public Health in Canada: A Report of the National Advisory Committee on SARS and Public Health* (Ottawa: Health Canada, 2003). At www.hc-sc.gc.ca/english/protection/warnings/sars/learning/EngSe30 on 10/26/2003; Ontario Expert Panel on SARS and Infectious Disease Control (David Walker, chair), *For the Public's Health: A Plan of Action* (Toronto: SARS Expert Panel Secretariat. Ontario. Ministry of Health and Long-Term Care, 2003). At www.health.gov.on.ca. The Independent SARS Commission (Justice Archie Campbell, chair), *SARS and Public Health in Ontario*, Interim Report (15 April 2004). At www.health.gov.on.ca/english/public/pub/ministry_reports/campbell04. Mr. Justice Archie Campbell, *SARS and Public Health Legislation*, Second Interim Report (5 April 2005).

[60]Sheela V. Basrur, Barbara Yaffe and Bonnie Henry, "SARS: A Local Public Health Perspective," *Canadian Journal of Public Health* 95 (January/February 2004):22-24.

[61]Colin D'Cunha, "SARS: Lessons Learned from a Provincial Perspective," *Canadian Journal of Public Health* 95 (January/February 2004):25-26.

[62]Carolyn Abraham and Caroline Alphonso, "Crossed Wires Put Toronto on Hit List," *Globe and Mail*, Thursday, 24 April 2003, pp. A1, A7; see also Danylo Hawaleshka, "SARS: Is this your Best Defence?" *Maclean's Magazine*, 14 April 2003, p. 24; Colin Freeze, "Commuters into Toronto Ride out Scare," *Globe and Mail*, Tuesday, 22 April 2003, p. A5; Jonathon Gatehouse, "SARS: Fear and Loathing of Toronto," *Maclean's Magazine*, 5 May 2003, pp. 19-22.

[63]"A Canadian Agency for Public Health: If Not Now, When? "Editorial, *Canadian Medical Association Journal* 169, no. 8 (2003); Wayne Kondro, "Public Health on the Installment Plan," *Canadian Medical Association Journal* 170, no. 9 (2004); Health Canada, News Release, "Government of Canada Announces Details of New Public Health Agency of Canada and Appoints Acting Chief Public Health Officer," 17 May 2004; Carolyn Bennett, "Building a National Public Health System, *Canadian Medical Association Journal* 170, no. 9 (2004).

[64]Richard Mackie, "Ontario to Put SARS Lessons into Practice," *Globe and Mail*, Wednesday, 23 June 2004, p. A9.

[65]André Picard, "Mommy, Are You Going to Die?" *Globe and Mail*, Saturday 5 April 2003, p. F5; Basrur, Yaffe and Henry, "SARS," p. 24. "In addition, attention to the so-called 'Recovery' phase usually does not make it onto anyone's radar screen, particularly once the pressure is on to revert to 'normal.' It takes time to recover from the stress of responding to an emergency situation, particularly one of the duration and magnitude of SARS. This must not be forgotten."

7

MAKING HISTORY: TB AND THE PUBLIC HEALTH LEGACY OF SARS IN CANADA

Georgina Feldberg

Like cities everywhere, Toronto has seen far worse than SARS in the past, and lived to tell the tale. Infectious diseases now barely remembered once felled thousands and helped shape public health care.[1]

When the family of Toronto's first (but as yet undiagnosed) SARS victim arrived at the emergency room of the Scarborough Grace Hospital, on 7 March 2003, the attending physician suspected that their coughing, fever, and shortness of breath were signs of tuberculosis (TB). Tuberculosis was a logical diagnosis. "We have a large immigrant population in this hospital, Chinese and Indian," Dr. Finkelstein observed, "and here everything is TB until proven otherwise."[2] The radiologist's interpretation of chest X-rays, taken the following day, supported a diagnosis of tuberculosis. However, Dr. Finkelstein had never previously seen a cluster of TB cases. His inquiry to Toronto Public Health soon confirmed that the city was confronting something quite different — a sudden outbreak of a newly emerging infection, SARS.

Over the course of the next months, SARS distinguished itself from TB in significant ways. Nonetheless, as SARS left a lasting impression on the public imagination and a deep imprint on health-care management and administration it continually mirrored the history of TB. SARS, like TB, is spread by sputum and coughing, and fear of infection transformed public behaviours. TB, like SARS, was often imported. SARS, like TB, took a heavy toll among health-care workers — both physicians and nurses. Both diseases shaped the public imagination, took an economic toll, and reconfigured health care. In 1924, threats of bovine and human tuberculosis prompted the government to form an Associate Committee on Tuberculosis Research, which metamorphosed into the Medical Research Council of Canada. The 2003 SARS outbreak prompted the Government of Canada to restructure public health, with an inquiry into the public health system and the establishment of a Public Health Agency, a minister of state for Public Health and a chief public health officer.[3]

Both diseases also *made* history. SARS, like tuberculosis, transformed the ways in which Canadians write and think about infections. More importantly, the ways in which journalists and others invoked history to talk about and explain SARS illustrated the important yet problematic role that history plays in the formation of Canadian health policy. "Policymakers at every level," writes historian Susan Reverby, "need a past as a touch stone ... To gain such a place, they often create the stories they want finding safety in uncomplicated historical narratives, journalistic accounts, or the mining of what historians have written to serve their purposes."[4] History, or stories from the past, became an important way in which public responses to SARS took shape. Yet, as Reverby, Fox, and other policy historians note, the public accounts emphasized only certain stories and episodes from the twentieth-century conquest of infections.[5] The "history" was partial and largely journalistic.

This chapter examines the ways in which Canadian newspapers invoked history, and relied on historians as experts, during the SARS epidemic. Appeals to history and historians, during these months, were unprecedented. In Canada, neither HIV/AIDS nor other infections provoked such historicizing. The historical accounts presented in newspapers are consequently important because they provide examples of the ways in which disease history is created for public purposes. However, newspapers also have critical implications for health policy. Successful programs of infection control rely on both the creation and the implementation of policy. They demand that the public both understand and comply with, or act on, policy recommendations. Yet, as feminist health critics have argued, perception gaps — vast differences in expectations — often impede the implementation of policy. Newspapers, which both shape and reflect popular knowledge, offer glimpses into those perception gaps. The choice of experts, examples, and stories allows us to consider the alternative histories that might have been told. Had newspapers and experts invoked the history of tuberculosis rather than plague, for example, the public response to infection control might have been quite different. An historically contingent comparison of TB and SARS prompts us to reflect on the ways in which we might frame our histories of disease so that "healthy public policy" balances health promotion initiatives with infection control.

TB proved to be the wrong medical diagnosis for the Tse family. Had Mr. Tse and his family indeed constituted a cluster of TB cases, it would have been medically more significant, if socially and politically less so. TB was, and continues to be, a major international killer. Unlike SARS, which emerged as a sudden outbreak that caused fewer than 1,000 deaths worldwide, one hundred in North America, tuberculosis was, and still is, one of the "great plagues." Paleontologic records suggest that TB has existed for centuries. Through the nineteenth century, and well into the twentieth century, it ranked as the leading cause of North American deaths. In the 1960s, after heart disease, cancer, automobile accidents, and what we call "lifestyle illnesses" replaced infections as the top causes of morbidity and mortality, tuberculosis and influenza remained the only infections among the most significant North American causes of death. TB affected more individuals than polio, measles, or more commonly feared infections. In 1949, as polio cases rose to the "epidemic" rate of 30 per 100,000 the TB case rate in the US exceeded 90 per 100,000, and TB claimed 4,382 Canadian lives.[6]

After World War II, hygienic measures (such as anti-spitting ordinances and dietary reforms, chemoprophylaxis (streptomycin, PAS, and isoniazid) and vaccination (BCG), combined to reduce mortality and morbidity to the extent that TB disappeared temporarily from public and medical memory. The demise was short lived. Within two decades, TB was back. It reappeared in the early 1980s, alongside HIV/AIDS, then continued to spread. By October 2000, Health Canada's *TB Watchdog* warned that TB was no longer in decline. Globally, the disease claimed 3 million lives each year; 3 million Canadians, or 10 percent of the national population, were TB carriers. A small fraction of carriers (2,000) would develop an active disease and fewer still would die, but Health Canada warned about deadly drug-resistant strains, prevalent in Europe and Asia, that air travel could easily spread.[7] Toronto, where the case rate of almost 500 per year was more than three times the national norm, was particularly vulnerable.[8] A disease of poverty that once prevailed among Inuit and First Nations' populations, TB is now an imported disease; new immigrants, those born outside Canada and have been in Canada for five years or less account for 87 percent of cases.[9]

SARS, in contrast, did not "fell thousands." It ultimately proved to be a minor "plague." Physicians breathed a sigh of relief in late March 2003, when the outbreak seemed to have run its course, and noted that SARS had a relatively low fatality rate. They even joked that it might be renamed MARS, with M standing for mild.[10] In strict terms of morbidity and mortality, SARS posed a far less threat than car accidents, cancers, or many other infections — malaria, influenza, and especially TB among them. By August 2003, when the second Toronto outbreak had long been officially over, there were 438 SARS cases and 44 deaths. Chagrined public health officers, such as Richard Schabas, former medical officer of health for the province of Ontario, noted that the toll of SARS paled when one considered that "as many people die of cigarette-related deaths every 8 hours." Schabas deemed SARS an "irritating blip" that distracted Canadians "from the problems that kill more people than SARS ever did."[11]

Tuberculosis ranks high among the diseases that Schabas urged Canadians to take seriously. Yet, today few Canadians know or worry about the dangers of contracting tuberculosis. Even as SARS renewed fears about public spitting, the threat of TB — spread most commonly through sputum — continued to fly below the radar. For example, in April 2004, when the newly elected mayor of Saskatoon, Saskatchewan, championed a bylaw that would fine those who spat in public $250, one city councillor worried that the city council would be laughed at as lunatic. "The big part isn't the spitting," he suggested, "it's the [public] urinating." With the confidence of most North Americans who have been insulated from infections, he expressed greater concern about the aesthetic problems of smell and conduct rather than the vehicles for disease communication.[12]

MAKING HISTORY: THE IMPACT AND SIGNIFICANCE OF SARS

SARS sensitized and mobilized Canadians because it made organizational, experiential, and interpretative history. Despite its limited duration and scope, the SARS outbreak profoundly "shape[d] public health care" and achieved what decades of federal and provincial health reform could not. It exposed the cracks in Canada's much prized health-care system, the decay of public health infrastructure, and the costs of emphasizing health promotion over disease prevention and control. Toronto's experience with SARS provoked the Government of Canada to review public health services and the split jurisdiction — federal, provincial, and local — for infectious disease. In May 2003, the federal minister of health established a National Advisory Committee on SARS, mandated to provide "third-party assessment of current public health efforts and lessons learned for ongoing infectious disease control."[13] SARS, and the assessment that followed, laid the foundation for a new Public Health Agency, ambivalently nicknamed "CDC North."

The panic that accompanied the SARS outbreak was unlike anything most Canadians had experienced. Fear, coupled with stigma and international travel sanctions, numbed Toronto's economy and forced the public and the three levels of Canadian government that share responsibility for public health (city, provincial, and federal) to reconsider the social and medical impacts of infections. Despite the reality that HIV and tuberculosis are prevalent in North American cities, most affluent North Americans have been insulated from, and hence feel immune to, the impacts of epidemics and contagion. Those older than 65 might remember polio outbreaks, diphtheria quarantines, tuberculosis sanatoria, or influenza scares, but the shadow of cancer and "lifestyle diseases" generally stretches much further than that cast by infections. Twenty-first century threats, bio-terrorism, then newly emerging infections, consequently fell on new soil and disrupted a social sense of well-being. "It all has the feel of a watershed moment," one Toronto reporter wrote. "For the most part, public health scourges were supposed to have died out in the West. Although much of the world suffers from malaria and tuberculosis, we felt immune. We thought we had beaten back disease, even kept a lid on HIV/AIDS, because of our affluence, science, and education."[14] Long after Toronto was SARS-free and the World Health Organization (WHO) travel ban lifted, Torontonians remembered SARS. In subways and public places, fear of infection persisted and throughout the summer and fall of 2003, people flinched each time someone coughed or sneezed. One year later, political scandals replaced illness in newspaper headlines, but an opinion piece in the Toronto *Globe and Mail* nonetheless used the spectre of SARS [though once again not TB] to denounce "horking" [public spitting].[15]

SARS made history in still another sense; it compelled Canadians to remember the past. During the early days of the outbreak, as physicians struggled to contain infection, reassure health-care workers and patients, and keep the city's economy on an even course, Canadians groped for historical precedents that would explicate, normalize, and reassure. Some of the groping for historical security was tangible. Not sure what else to do, physicians and public health officials resorted to quarantine, a venerable if antiquarian practice that once again became the best way of controlling infection. The resurrection of outdated but historically tested disease-control measures also encouraged patients, practitioners, and the media to think historically. Precedents from the history of public health, along with historians of medicine, briefly gained prominence as journalists sought academics who could discuss influenza, plague, smallpox, typhoid, and other "historical" epidemic infections. Readers of Toronto's daily newspapers, *The Star, The Globe and Mail,* and the *National Post,* quickly received a crash course in the history of medicine as they were overwhelmed with articles that invoked historical precedents. Reports and editorials introduced Canadians to Hippocrates, the plague, and most frequently, the 1918 Spanish Flu. A search for references to SARS and history/historian/historical/ or historically, found in Toronto newspapers published during the period of the outbreak, produced over 300 hits in the *Toronto Star,* over 100 in *The Globe and Mail,* and 231 in the *National Post.* History and policy became intertwined as precedents were constructed, even distorted, to give SARS meaning.

The press coverage of SARS often used fear mongering.[16] Journalists, academics, policy analysts, and the public alike seized upon SARS to air their anxieties about the collapse of scientific, hospital-based medicine. Headlines proclaimed "Invisible army shakes faith in science" or "Microbes Scary."[17] "In the modern world, people don't worry much about becoming a lion's dinner or their children being carried off by wolves," science reporter Stephen Strauss wrote in *The Globe and Mail,* "but microbes — tiny rapacious multitudinous microbes — scare everyone."[18] Some made the stretch to "Bio-terrorism, are we ready for a germ war?" and asked, "If SARS has stricken our health-care and emergency systems, what would we do in a deliberate attack?"[19] Others focused on the need for health-care reform. Jamie Swift, longtime labour analyst, took the opportunity to denounce decades of government cuts to health-care financing and to make the case for improved home care.[20] Popularist Andrew Nikiforuk reminded readers of *The Globe and Mail* that SARS highlighted "the shoddy state of infection control in our hospitals," which "thanks to medical cost-cutters and promiscuous antibiotic use" had become "microbial feedlots."[21]

Yet, perhaps because they were written in the heat of panic, during the hot days of the outbreak, newspapers sought out historians and invoked history to help Canadians understand how and why we had managed to conquer other infections. At a time when Canadians faced the fearful unknown, history provided security and comfort. "To get a sense of the context for how the current war against severe acute respiratory syndrome is likely to go, the past provides a useful context," Stephen Straus advised.[22] "The SARS epidemic has some of the traits of plague," the *National Post* reminded its readers, but "Thucydides, the great Athenian historian, was infected with the plague of 430 BC and lived to tell the tale."[23] Tara Perkins, writing in *The Globe and Mail*, proposed that SARS might not be so new and unknown. Noting that SARS shared many symptoms with the case of Hermocrates that Hippocrates had described, she asked, "And what was the great man's diagnosis? Some new bug from China's Guangdong Province perhaps?"[24] Other articles reassured readers that there were "encouraging differences" between SARS and the 1918 influenza pandemic."[25] Historian Michael Bliss reminded readers that his book *Plague!*, a description of Montreal's experience with smallpox, "ended on a positive note because smallpox never recurred on such a scale in any Western city."[26] Still others drew comparisons to the eradication of infections that followed the bacteriologic and chemotherapeutic revolutions of the late nineteenth and early twentieth centuries.

SARS AND THE LEGACY OF TB

The uses of history in newspaper coverage of SARS reflected and reinforced perception gaps about the conquest of infection, as references to tuberculosis, few though they were, illustrate. Appeals to *Clio medica* continued long after the SARS outbreak had subsided. In October 2003, the newsletter of Toronto's West Park Health Centre, a reconfigured TB sanatorium, invoked history in its publicity campaign. Affirming "The Power of Community" the hospital asserted that:

> When SARS hit Toronto, the people of West Park pulled together. Almost one hundred years ago, West Park Health Centre (formerly The Toronto Free Hospital for the Consumptive Poor and the Weston Sanatorium) offered new hope for victims of a frightening and poorly understood disease. Despite the risk of infection, physicians, nurses and others worked together to care for patients

with tuberculosis, and to expand knowledge of the disease.... This spring, West
Park again opened its arms to the victims of another frightening and poorly
understood disease. This time it was Severe Acute Respiratory Syndrome
(SARS).[27]

West Park's statement exemplified efforts to use history to reassure. It prom-
ised that Canadians had both learned and profited from the past, that they would
build upon historical knowledge to ensure that SARS was eradicated, and that
like TB, SARS would be conquered.

However, West Park exists as an isolation facility today precisely because TB has not been conquered. The hospital's appeal to history is puzzling,
since rather than reassuring readers and potential donors, the historical comparisons might easily have drawn attention to the failure of tuberculosis-control
efforts. The identification of the bacterial source of TB did not allow physicians
to eradicate it. In fact, scientific management, long-term chemoprophylaxis,
helped produce drug-resistant forms.

The apparent failure of TB-control programs lends historical meaning
to the SARS outbreak *and* provides the most compelling application of history
to public practice and policy. Yet, the press did not invoke this history, nor was
the policy potential drawn out.

Tuberculosis, as it exists in drug-resistant forms today, should be frightening. However, during the early years of the twentieth century, TB was
pervasive and prevalent but, contrary to what West Park suggested, it was less
"frightening" and "poorly understood" than commonplace. Everyone knew
someone who had TB. Many had it themselves. Most knew those who lived
with the disease, or recovered. As with SARS, where 90 percent of cases were
health-care workers, TB was so pervasive that few physicians or nurses escaped infection.[28] But in contrast to SARS, doctors and nurses figured
prominently in narratives of both illness and recovery. Allen Krause and Edward
Livingston Trudeau (founder of the American Sanatorium movement) were
among those who fell ill, recovered, and went back to work. Confident that a
diagnosis of tuberculosis need not be a death sentence, they incorporated programs of occupational therapy and rehabilitation into the treatment regimens
they prescribed. As founders of sanatoria, they described their institutions as
"educational centres" or "abodes for reconstruction, education and rehabilitation" where consumptives could be taught to live with their disease.[29] Tubercular

physicians' affirmations of the ways patients could learn to manage sputum, live productively and not infect others were partly self-serving; the affirmations enabled tuberculous physicians to resume their own work unafraid that they would tax their own health or endanger their patients.

Assurances that health-care workers need not fear tuberculosis patients, and that the tuberculous could safely undertake health-care work, also provided a route for rehabilitation. Rather than fearing infection or facing unemployment, patients might find work helping others overcome TB. This opportunity was particularly useful to tuberculous women. Often advised not to marry, work in factories, or take up domestic and service positions, these women had limited opportunities. Tuberculosis nursing came to be deemed "the most favorable kind of occupation for such patients who must earn their own living."[30]

By the early decades of the twentieth century, folk wisdom, and the scientific knowledge that followed Robert Koch's identification of the tubercle bacillus in 1882, combined to make tuberculosis, or consumption, seem manageable. As Allen K. Krause, professor of pathology at Johns Hopkins University and director of the Kenneth Dows Tuberculosis Laboratory noted in 1918: "Becoming enthusiastic because of several remarkable discoveries made in rapid succession we began to make claims. Made bold by unexpected success, we began to predict. We could cure tuberculosis ... so flushed were we in the first days of our new knowledge that we set the date for the disappearance of tuberculosis ... the banners that flaunted 'No More Tuberculosis by 1915.'"[31] The banners and predictions were wrong. TB persisted, but North Americans would believe they could eradicate it again, and again, and again.

The role that knowledge of bacteria and bacteriocides played in TB's decline remains ambiguous; tuberculous mortality and morbidity began to fall well before specific antibiotics or vaccines became available. The role played by bacterial infection in disease causation was also debatable. Before Robert Koch identified the tubercle bacillus, in 1882, few Europeans or North Americans believed the disease to be contagious. Instead, they classified TB as diathetic or constitutional, thereby assigning responsibility to behaviour and inherent physical predisposistion. Long after 1882, North Americans continued to believe that TB was a disease of both seed and soil.[32] Leading physicians, Edward Livingston Trudeau, Allan Krause, and even Robert Koch, held tubercle bacilli only partial responsibility for tuberculosis. "For the occurrence of tuberculosis in any given case," physicians repeatedly insisted, "two factors are necessary, the proper soil and the infectious agent."[33]

Physicians did not immediately embrace Koch's findings, and they did not immediately assume that knowledge of the bacteriologic causes of disease would allow them to control infections. They remained circumspect. Even after 1882, medical opinion agreed that tuberculosis was not highly contagious and that exposure to the tubercle bacillus, or infection, would not necessarily result in disease. Tuberculin testing, introduced during the early decades of the twentieth century, reinforced this, demonstrating that a positive reaction, indicative of infection, was not necessarily proof of disease. Moreover, exposure did not necessarily produce infection. Those who lived well might come into regular contact with tubercle bacilli but not fall ill.

Throughout the first half of the twentieth century, local and national public health agencies, and the National Tuberculosis Association repeatedly issued bulletins that reminded Americans that TB was communicable rather than contagious. They reassured the public that "careful" consumptives posed little threat to their families or communities. In schools, sanatoria, and communities, concerted educational campaigns taught consumptives — sometimes in colourful terms — how to live safely and not to share their germs with others. Quarantine, a major feature of the SARS epidemic, did not play a significant role in the control of TB because North Americans did not believe that the tuberculous posed a general threat. Public health and social service agencies used quarantine as a last resort, when the individual would not manage his sputum correctly and responsibly, not because tuberculosis posed a danger in and of itself.[34]

Buoyed by the successes of mid-century campaigns against infections, later histories recast responses to bacteria, particularly tubercle bacillus, to affirm the successes of a bacteriologic revolution.[35] History was reshaped to erase the ambivalence and circumspection that characterized many physicians' initial reactions to the identification of specific "germs." When TB mortality and morbidity declined significantly during the 1950s and 1960s, physicians and historians alike cast TB into an emblem of successful scientific medicine. They upheld it as one of the triumphs of the "bacteriologic, immunologic and chemotherapeutic period."[36] That historical rewriting is reflected in West Park's statements, and in the journalism that contextualized SARS with laments about the decline of modern medicine. Historical reframing produced the faith in biomedicine, reliance on its interventions, and disappointment in its shortcomings, that became so evident in the panic that accompanied the SARS outbreak. As they struggled to understand and control SARS, physicians and lay sources alike voiced betrayal. "Last year, a deadly virus came upon us by stealth," David Walker, dean of health sciences at Queen's University noted that:

> The world seems to have become a more hostile place. Just as we are attempting to come to terms with the horrendous effects of terrorist acts we find that our traditional and oft-forgotten adversaries, microbes, have awoken with renewed vigour and threat. Around the world, HIV causes a disease that decimates populations; tuberculosis, now often resistant to drugs, has returned in force, while old foes such as malaria kill hundreds of humans each day. Hospital-acquired infections cause thousands of deaths, the safety of our water supply has been challenged, a mosquito bite can transmit West Nile virus, and concerns about North American cattle are in the news.[37]

SARS, BSE, avian flu, and other newly emerging infections seem frightening because they appear to shatter the historical record, but in fact they do not. Instead, they invite us to remember the more temperate, if less valiant and reassuring, history of TB control. History, properly remembered and applied to newly emerging infections, prompts us to reconsider the role that *both* soil and seed played in public health campaigns and to champion the reintegration of public health and public welfare.

RESISTING INFECTION: THE SOCIAL SIDE OF PUBLIC HEALTH

SARS highlighted the numerous cracks in the Canadian health-care system. As many have noted, it drew attention to the ways in which underfunding, privatization, and employment have eroded publicly funded Canadian hospital care. SARS is important for another, less recognized reason: SARS highlighted the costs of a conceptual shift in public health that dichotomized, or strictly differentiated, efforts to eradicate bacteria from public interventions that acted to improve the human soil. In the 1970s, the focus of western public health moved from infections to chronic conditions. Public health initiatives began to emphasize the transformation of behaviours (e.g., smoking, high-fat diets, inadequate exercise) linked to chronic illness. As campaigns to prevent infectious disease took second place to health promotion, the infrastructure needed to combat infection crumbled.[38]

The public sense of what infection means also changed. When, or if, they think about germs, most modern North Americans turn to vaccines, drugs or cleaning products as their first line of defence. The uses of history in newspaper stories about SARS reinforced these assumptions and behaviours. Yet, other stories might have been told. These stories would have highlighted the early twentieth-century activists who framed official tuberculosis-control policy with a broader view. The alternative history would recognize a range of activists who underscored the need for chemotherapy, behavioural change (e.g., anti-spitting), *and* improved standards of living. It would emphasize the ways in which antituberculosis initiatives recognized the dual roles of seed and soil, and the ways they intertwined campaigns of healthy living with campaigns of social reform. Alongside measures to control bacteria, public health campaigns to combat TB promoted diet, hygiene, and exercise. They also underscored the social and economic origins of vulnerability to infections. Writing in the 1920s, Krause located the causes of disease in "the cities, the streets, the houses, and backyards, the rooms in which we live and move, the baths, the windows, the stoves, the furniture, the clothing, the space, air, and sunlight which people may or may not have," and in "the environment of occupations."[39] In 1946, the United States Public Health Service (USPHS) argued that the best means of controlling TB in the general population was, "improvement of living conditions and general health" alongside measures that reduced infection, such as anti-spitting ordinances and dietary reform.[40] Through the first half of the twentieth century, institutional and non-institutional tuberculosis-control programs alike recognized the links between tuberculosis and economic vulnerability. They adopted a rhetoric of rehabilitation and reform that they combined with occupational skills training. Tubercular patients learned how to safely manage sputum so that they might resume regular activity. They also received occupational therapy to facilitate a speedy and sustained return to productive work.[41] As late as 1955, leading American public health officials congratulated TB hospitals for "providing extra-medical services ... namely education, diversional and occupational therapy, counselling, testing, vocational guidance, training, job placement."[42]

The modern transformation of public health has, often unwittingly, pitted "lifestyle" diseases against infection control. If the focus on chronic disease allowed the public to forget infections, it also allowed them to forget that the pillars of health promotion and disease prevention are not necessarily incompatible. It erased public awareness that infections, like TB, still require both a seed *and* a receptive soil, that welfare and social spending promote public health, and that "health promoting" behaviours — diet or even simple hand-washing — can also limit infection by preventing the spread or the impact of microbes. Newspaper coverage of SARS built on this narrow historical vision.

Tuberculosis is a disease of the physically and socially vulnerable in a way that SARS, at least in Canada, was not.[43] Diet, hygiene, exercise, and economic status continue to play a significant role in rendering individuals resistant to TB; we do not know their role in the etiology of SARS. Nonetheless, as Canadians remake public health in the shadow of SARS, the history of TB, and of its control, provide opportunities for reflection. These histories ask us to reconsider the ways in which we distinguish lifestyle risks from infections, and they prompt us to reflect on the primacy and power we accord microbes, vaccinations, and antibiotics. Post-SARS, Canadians anxiously await the next superbug (BSE, or avian flu, or West Nile) and they place their faith in tests, vaccines, drugs, and communication mechanisms that will allow for effective identification and speedy "emergency response."

Yet, the 2003 influenza season, laden with recent memories of SARS, made it clear that vaccination is not a public health cure-all. The virulence and onset of the 2003 influenza season seemed to herald an epidemic even more forbidding than SARS. Bug-shy Ontarians lined up for hours, in clinics, malls, and even grocery stores, to receive flu shots, indisputably a strong defence against illness. However, the crowds awaiting flu shots arguably also increased the risk of infection.

Ads in the subways suggested that vaccination was a form of civic responsibility. These ads did not pay equal service to the promotion of behaviours — washing hands, not spitting, covering the mouth or nose, or staying out of crowds — that are also historic and tested methods of infection control. Policy attended to vaccination, but not to social programs of entitlement to sick leave, a form of voluntary quarantine for those who are unwell or who act as caregivers to sick dependents, that can also limit the spread of infection. Nonetheless, as Canada laments the erosion of its public health system and seeks renewal, discussion of such social and economic policy change remains in the background while military style "emergency response preparedness" moves to the foreground.

"Public health must be invigorated and resuscitated as a societal priority,"[44] David Walker wrote in his capacity as chair of the Ontario Expert Panel on SARS and Infectious Disease Control. Physician-historian David Naylor, then dean of the Medical School at the University of Toronto and chair of the federal government's National Advisory Committee on SARS, concurred. They, and other commissioners who examined the state of Canadian public health post-SARS identified the need and made a compelling case for infection-control networks, protocols, and disease surveillance plans, supported by information technology. However, the history of tuberculosis, applied to SARS, serves as a reminder that public health needs more than anti-microbial measures. In the past, attacks on microbes alone did not conquer infectious disease. The history of tuberculosis reminds us of, and points us toward, the reintegration of the social, political, and the biomedical within public health initiatives.

NOTES

[1] Elaine Carey, "The Survivor of a Thousand Plagues," *Toronto Star*, 26 April 2003, p. B04.

[2] Carolyn Abraham, "The SARS Outbreak: How a Deadly Disease Made its Way to Canada, *The Globe and Mail*, 29 March 2003.

[3] C. David Naylor *et al.*, *Learning from SARS: Renewal of Public Health in Canada, A Report of the National Advisory Committee on SARS and Public Health.* (Ottawa: National Advisory Committee on SARS and Public Health, 2003) p. 2; Health Canada, Public Health Agency. At www.hc-sc.gc.ca.

[4] Susan Reverby, "Thinking Through the Body and the Body Politic," in *Women Health and Nation: Canada and the United States since 1945,* ed. G. Feldberg *et al.* (Montreal and Kingston: McGill-Queen's University Press, 2003), p. 406.

[5] Daniel Fox, "History and Health Policy: An Autobiographical Note on the Decline of Historicism," *Journal of Social History* 18 (Spring 1986):349-64.

[6] In Canada, TB mortality was almost 50/1000,000, higher in the Indian or First Nations' populations. See J.G. Wherrett, *Miracle of the Empty Beds: A History of Tuberculosis in Canada* (Toronto: University of Toronto Press, 1977), pp. 251-52. In the US, overall TB mortality was 28/100,000 with immigrants, Native and African Americans having both higher incidence and mortality. See United States Bureau of the Census, *Historical Statistics of the United States: Colonial Times to 1970* (New York: Cambridge University Press, 1997), Vol. 1, pp. 58-77.

[7] Health Canada, *TB Watchdog*, October 2000.

[8] City of Toronto, Public Health, *Status of Health in 2001* (Toronto: City of Toronto Public Health, 2001), TB pamphlets.

[9] City of Toronto: *Status of Health.*

[10]Abraham, "Status of SARS."

[11]Richard Schabas, "Don't Cry Wolf on Every Flu, " *The Globe and Mail*, 2 February 2004, p. A11.

[12]Graeme Smith, "Canada's Craziest Mayor Earns New Title: Mr. Clean," *The Globe and Mail*, 10 April 2004, p. F3.

[13]Naylor, *Learning from SARS*.

[14]"Confronting the Perils of a Shrinking World," *The Globe and Mail*, 28 March 2003.

[15]Cecily Ross, "And Another Thing ... Public Spitting," *The Globe and Mail*, 22 May 2004, p. M7.

[16]Daniel Drache and David Clifton, "Media Coverage of the 2003 Toronto SARS Outbreak: A Report on the Role of the Press in a Public Crisis." Presentation to the Robarts Centre for Canadian Studies, 29 October 2003. Unpublished paper; see also Schabas, "Don't Cry Wolf."

[17]Jim Coyle "Invisible Army Shakes Faith in Science," *Toronto Star*, 29 March 2003, p. A 04.

[18]Stephen Straus, "Microcosm-Microbes are Scary," *The Globe and Mail*, 5 April 2003.

[19]Donald Avery, "Bioterrorism: Are We Ready for a Germ War?" *The Globe and Mail*, 3 April 2003.

[20]Jamie Swift, " Home Care Now More than Ever," *The Globe and Mail*, 24 April 2003.

[21]Andrew Nikiforuk, "Past Plagues are Prologue: Epidemics Always Teach us Something," *The Globe and Mail*, 26 April 2003.

[22]Straus, "Microcosm-Microbes,"

[23]Gerald Owen, "A Journal of the Plague Years: If You Think SARS is Bad, Ever Heard of the Black Death?" *National Post*, 5 April 2003.

[24]Tara Perkins, "Mystery Illness: Settlers Quarantined to Contain Disease," *The Globe and Mail*, 23 March 2003.

[25]Anne Milroy, "1918 Redux? SARS Shares Many Frightening Similarities with the Spanish Flu Pandemic that Killed 20 Million Around the World, but the Differences Between the Outbreaks are what Might Save Us," *The Globe and Mail*, 5 April 2003.

[26]Michael Bliss, "When Deadly Viruses Burn in our Cities," *National Post*, 14 April 2003.

[27]West Park Hospital, "The Power of Community," *Newsletter*, Fall 2003.

[28]Abraham, "Status of SARS"; Naylor, *Learning from SARS*.

[29]Allan K. Krause, "Antituberculosis Measures," in *Rest and Other Things: A Little Book of Plain Talks on Tuberculosis Problems* (Baltimore, MD: Williams & Wilkins Co., 1923), p. 77; Julius Wilson, "Daily Sanatorium Routine was the Treatment," *American Lung Association Bulletin* (March 1982), p. 8. See also Georgina Feldberg, *Disease and Class: Tuberculosis and the Shaping of Modern North American Society* (New Brunswick, NJ: Rutgers University Press, 1995).

[30]Philadelphia Hospital, "Circular of Information for the Special Course on the Nursing of Tuberculosis," Walsh Papers, Vol. 2 (Philadelphia, PA: College of Physicians of Philadelphia, n.d.).

[31]Allen K. Krause, "Antituberculosis Measures," reprinted from the *American Review of Tuberculosis*, December 1918 in Krause, *Rest and Other Things*, p. 64.

[32]Feldberg, *Disease and Class*, esp. ch. 2.

[33]"Proceedings of the Ohio Medical Society, June 1884," *Cincinnati Lancet and Clinic* 12 (1884):741.

[34]The circumspection that physicians, and especially public health workers, displayed about the role of bacilli and bacteriocides in infectious disease control characterized not only TB but also other diseases, like polio and typhoid. See Naomi Rogers, *Disease and Dirt: Polio Before FDR* (New Brunswick, NJ: Rutgers University Press, 1992); Judith Walzer Leavitt, *Typhoid Mary: Captive to the Public's Health* (Boston: Beacon Press, 1996).

[35]See, for example, George Rosen, "The Bacteriologic, Immunologic and Chemotherapeutic Period, 1875–1950," *Bulletin of the New York Academy of Medicine* 40 (1964):483-94. For further discussion, see Feldberg, *Disease and Class*.

[36]Rosen, "Bacteriologic, Immunologic and Chemotherapeutic Period."

[37]David Walker, "Are We Ready for the Next Killer Bug?" *The Globe and Mail*, 13 January 2004, p. A21.

[38]Walker, "Are We Ready?"; Naylor, *Learning from SARS*.

[39]Allen K. Krause, *Environment and Resistance to Tuberculosis* (Baltimore, MD: Williams & Wilkins, 1923), p. 8.

[40]"Present Policy of the American Trudeau Society on BCG Vaccination," *American Review of Tuberculosis* 57 (1948):545.

[41]Feldberg, *Disease and Class*, pp. 93-100, 106-07.

[42]Hermann Hilleboe and Robert Plunkett, "Division of Tuberculosis Control State of New York to County, City and District Health Officers: Current Concepts in the Drug Treatment of Non-Hospitalized Tuberculosis Patients," National Archives of the United States, 9 March 1955, RG 90-62A-177, box 7.

[43]For further discussion of TB, and its impacts in the late twentieth century, see Paul Farmer, *Infections and Inequalities: The Modern Plagues* (Berkley: University of California Press, 1999).

[44]Walker, "Are We Ready?"

8

SARS in the Light of Sexually Transmitted Diseases *and* AIDS

Jay Cassel

I come from a place that taxi drivers call the "fruit basket," locals call the "ghetto," and the City of Toronto calls Church-Wellesley. When SARS struck in March 2003 the locals were preoccupied with another issue: "barebacking." Only the police ride horses in downtown Toronto. In the gay ghetto barebacking means anal sex without the use of a condom. Word on the street was that many gay men had sex occasionally without a condom. Some gay men did it by preference many times. Recently there was a major outbreak of syphilis in Montreal and Toronto. Nationally, the number of HIV-positive tests was rising. The AIDS Committee of Toronto was sufficiently concerned that it undertook a public health survey of sexual practices. It confirmed the word on the street.[1]

I am old enough to remember when men sat on the Steps, a well-known public space in front of the Second Cup at Church and Wellesley, with Kaposi's sarcoma on their faces. I remember holding the emaciated hand of a 29-year old friend, looking into his sunken eyes, and hearing him say "I'm afraid to die." He was not alone.

The gay community organized. They learned everything they could about AIDS and opportunistic infections. They pressed doctors to learn more and manage cases better. There would be no meek acceptance of medical authority! The community pressed the federal and provincial governments to release promising drugs. The gay community turned to science and they demanded a solution. They also demanded a role in formulating the solution.

In the midst of the barebacking issue came news of a new disease. No one knew the cause, but it killed people — fast. Toronto turned to science and looked for action. It soon emerged that we were dealing with a coronavirus, another disease for which a drug would be hard to develop. But like HIV, the coronavirus passed with difficulty, and the risky practices were soon identified.[2] The public health system activated its infection prevention regulations for the public and for health-care workers. The results appeared in the graph presented in the chapter by Dr. James Young.

During the 1980s, I wrote a history of the first campaign against Sexually Transmitted Disease (STD).[3] Basically, in the nineteenth century, doctors slowly worked out the nature of the diseases, then in the early twentieth century they developed diagnostic tests and a more effective treatment. It turned out that gonorrhea and syphilis were alarmingly prevalent in Canada. During the First World War, the Canadian Expeditionary Force had the highest incidence of infection of any army in Europe. The Canadian Army Medical Corps was obliged to organize a campaign to deal with the problem. This became the model for an STD campaign for the general public, which was launched in 1918.

The Canadian STD program had five components: medical measures – government funded diagnosis and treatment available free of charge to all Canadians; social work – contact tracing and public health nursing to ensure compliance with treatment; regulation of conduct – public health regulations to restrict activities of infected individuals; epidemiological work – statistics to trace patterns of infection and assess the progress of measures; education – to inform the medical profession and the general public about the diseases, their prevention, and what to do if infected. The medical measures remained in place from 1918 to the present, making STD an important early stage in the development of medicare.

The Americans went about things differently. Allan Brandt, the leading American historian of STDs argued: "in its transformation from a biological entity to a social symbol, [sexually transmitted disease] has defied control ... so long as these social uses of the diseases have dominated medical and public approaches, therapeutic approaches have necessarily remained secondary."[4] The Canadian story clearly did not fit that analysis closely.

Allan Brandt and I did agree on a number of points. We argued for candour in public discussions and in education about disease, sexual practices, and methods of prevention. Both of us were critical of the emphasis on "abstinence," "sexual continence," and "sex within marriage," which was always the leading line in American and Canadian education programs, although that was not the only message delivered to Canadians, especially in the armed forces! We argued that much could be accomplished by making condoms freely available, and that a thoroughly informed public would modify behaviour more effectively and in ways more easily tolerated by the common person than the approach favoured by the Women's Christian Temperance Union.

At the high-water mark of the AIDS crisis, I wrote an essay called "Making Canada Safe for Sex" in a collection edited by Dr. David Naylor, who would later chair the National Advisory Committee on SARS.[5] I noted that the three STD campaigns in Canadian history (World War I and after; World War II; and the one touched off by the sexual revolution of the later 1960s and 1970s) all had similar patterns: initial success, a period when results flattened out, and then a revival of the problem.

I concluded that the reason we could not resolve the problem of STD was the complex interplay of five factors: the nature of the diseases themselves, the limitations of medical remedies, social processes influencing public health programs and public perceptions, personal needs and psychological states, and the economics of health care and limited funding by governments. I also stressed the need for programs and regulations that were "sensitive to human realities" — frank acknowledgement of sexual diversity, candid communication and education, and feasible behavioural recommendations.

Underneath the nicely turned phrases was an academic's belief in education: work constructively with people's minds and marvels will follow: "Wisdom and Knowledge Shall be the Stability of Thy Times." Barebacking blows a big hole in that argument.

In my earlier writing, I praised the gay community for adopting just what Allan Brandt and I favoured — very candid education programs accepting a wide range of sexual practices as well as information geared to help the public make informed choices. Leading the way was the AIDS Committee of Toronto. They produced erotic safer-sex posters. They published explicit educational pamphlets. The adult film industry made films with condoms clearly visible — the action looked natural and hot, giving the impression that condoms were great, a part of the action, just like lubing up.

By 2003, I had heard from men that the images were artificially blissful (what a surprise!) and not everyone had sex that way. The committee became concerned. The survey they had conducted not only assessed practice, but attitudes as well. Researchers found that barebacking was done by men who were well-informed. They knew about AIDS, the limitations of drugs, and the risk levels of different activities.

People in the ghetto came up with several reasons why men were not always taking precautions.[6] The "cocktail" (combined drug therapy) diminished our fear of disease. With no Kaposi's sarcoma on the Steps, the horror of AIDS was out of sight. Sometimes HIV-positive men chose to have sex with other HIV-positive men. Sometimes passions overrode other considerations. Unlike the porn stars in gay videos, many men found it difficult to maintain an erection with a condom on. They tried various tricks to stay hard, but still there was something deflating about using condoms. During the First and Second World Wars, soldiers did not adhere closely to preventive measures. You don't have to be gay in the twenty-first century to slack off on prevention!

Even in the 1980s we said behaviour modification was difficult to maintain, and so it was best to work on the truly important changes, rather than try to get people to transform their lives. The gay community was supposed to be a great example of the wisdom of that approach. However, the history of past STD campaigns should have made us wary. People like Allan Brandt and myself criticized the way STD was used to enforce a certain conduct and a certain lifestyle (monogamy within heterosexual marriage). I would not change my position today, but I do note with dismay that getting people to modify their behaviour in face of a serious threat is difficult.

Slacking off on prevention is not unique to STD. The parallels during the SARS crisis are striking. Late in April 2003, Toronto hospitals eased off on infection-control precautions. Then on 23 May, just after the World Health Organization declared Toronto free of local transmission, we faced the stinging embarrassment of a new outbreak of SARS that went on for another month.[7] Later in 2003, I noticed that masks and hand-washing were sometimes ignored, especially by visitors to hospitals, despite signs urging people to wash. Mask boxes went away, and alcohol washes dried up. At one hospital I visited in January 2004, classic SARS measures were not reintroduced despite an influenza outbreak, and visitors did not heed signs urging them to wash their hands.

Early in the SARS crisis there was criticism of health-care workers who failed to follow guidelines for dealing with certain types of cases.[8] Many people picked up on the story of the nurse who rode the GO train between Toronto and Burlington, twice, while symptomatic.[9] Then a doctor at Sunnybrook Medical Health Centre went to a funeral, with symptoms of SARS. When he was placed in quarantine he was incensed and told the *Toronto Star* "I am a health-care professional. I would not knowingly put people at risk."[10] Evidently health-care workers felt at liberty to assess when public health regulations should apply to them. Experience in the STD, AIDS, and SARS campaigns shows that individuals do make calculations based on personal considerations that can lead them to depart from what others have objectively established is the best conduct in a public health crisis.

At the height of the AIDS crisis, the gay community demanded a lot of the government. It demanded a lot of medical practitioners. The dynamics of authority shifted. But the community also demanded a lot of its own members. We were supposed to be informed. We were supposed to act responsibly. Our health was our own affair. We would not just rely on the doctors. Somehow, it has left us thinking that we should assess the situation and determine our conduct as we see fit.

One AIDS Committee of Toronto researcher suggested a change in the message from "Take Care of Yourself" to "Take Care of Each Other."[11] The old issues, familiar to physicians and activists in the earlier STD campaigns, are still before us: compliance with recommended behaviour modifications and compliance with treatment regimens. I have grown wary of the easy answers of the common-sense conservatives as well as the certitudes of the left. What I have presented here is the first draft of a revision. In the light and darkness of SARS and AIDS, I am changing my view of the history of epidemics.

NOTES

[1]Barry Adam, Winston Husbands, James Murray and John Maxwell, *Renewing HIV Prevention for Gay and Bisexual Men: A Research Report on Safer Sex Practices among High-Risk Men and Men in Couples in Toronto* (Toronto, 2003).

[2]C. David Naylor *et al.*, *Learning from SARS: Renewal of Public Health in Canada, A Report of the National Advisory Committee on SARS and Public Health* (Ottawa: National Advisory Committee on SARS and Public Health, 2003) summarizes knowledge about the virus. Ch. 2 presents a chronological history of the SARS outbreak.

[3]Jay Cassel, *The Secret Plague: Venereal Disease in Canada, 1838-1939* (Toronto: University of Toronto Press, 1987).

[4]Allan M. Brandt, *No Magic Bullet: A Social History of Venereal Disease in the United States since 1880* (New York and Oxford: Oxford University Press, 1985), pp. 5, 6.

[5]Jay Cassel, "Making Canada Safe for Sex: Government and the Problem of Sexually Transmitted Disease in the Twentieth Century" in *Canadian Health Care and the State,* ed. C. David Naylor (Montreal and Kingston: McGill-Queen's University Press, 1992), pp. 141-92.

[6]This summary is based on my own conversations, numerous articles in the gay media, and the findings in Adam *et al., Renewing HIV Prevention.*

[7]Naylor *et al., Learning from SARS*, pp. 27, 38-42. "New SARS Fears Put 1,000 in Quarantine," *Toronto Star*, 24 May 2003, p. A1. "Thousands Caught up in SARS Crackdown," *Toronto Star*, 27 May 2003, p. A1. "Nurse Faces Second Quarantine – SARS Restrictions Were Eased too Soon She Says," *Toronto Star*, 28 May 2003, p. A8. Political pressure to return to normal was intense: "Ottawa Tries to Ease Toronto's Black Eye," *The Globe and Mail*, 24 April 2003, p. A1. *Globe* coverage was preoccupied with the implications for business.

[8]"Hospitals Blamed in Crisis," *Toronto Star*, 12 April 2003, p. A1.

[9]"Sick Nurse Sparks Alert for GO Riders," *Toronto Star*, 21 April 2003, p. A1; "Commuter Alert Opens New Phase in Battle," *The Globe and Mail*, 21 April 2003, p. A1.

[10]"Accused Doctor Angry," *Toronto Star,* 22 April 2003, pp. A1 and A8; "York Public Health Still Upset with Doctor Who Has Illness," *Toronto Star*, 23 April 2003, p. A8.

[11]James Murray, "The Bare Facts" *fab* [sic]18 Dec 2003, pp. 20-23.

Part III

PUBLIC POLICY IN THE AFTERMATH OF SARS

9

INTRODUCTION TO ECONOMIC ISSUES IN EPIDEMIOLOGY AND PUBLIC POLICY

Arthur Sweetman

E pidemics have substantial economic implications, and addressing epidemics has substantial economic motivation. The SARS epidemic has brought these ideas to the fore, and much attention is being paid by the press, think tanks, academia, and government to economic and governance issues in the preparation for future public health crises. Somewhat more recently the threat from avian flu has served to increase the attention paid to this area. These events have stimulated the subfield of economic epidemiology, which considers these topics, but has only begun to develop in the last decade or so. Much is yet to be learned about the relevant economic and governance issues, and a more balanced perspective is required than that provided in the heat of the moment during, or shortly after, a crisis when analyses are often undertaken. The goal of this chapter is to provide a brief and intuitive introduction to economic issues related to epidemics and allied public health issues, with some discussion of their public policy implications and the interaction between government and private actions. Three broad topics will be addressed in turn. First, I will review recent contributions that look at behavioural responses to epidemiological threats. This research approach looks at rational responses to epidemics by both individuals and collectives (especially governments); it considers the implications of strategic action in the face of an infectious threat. The second topic looks at the cost of infection, with a focus on the traditional economic notion of externalities. Globalization, in its various forms, adds greater relevance to some aspects of the costs of infection. Finally, I will look at the trade-offs inherent in public policy decision-making in the preparation for epidemics and in public health initiatives. Overlaying these three areas is the role of information.

BEHAVIOURAL RESPONSES

In the last decade, economic epidemiology research has started to look more carefully not only at how patterns of behaviour affect disease occurrence, but also at the feedback between disease prevalence and changes in behaviour. It is a move from traditional dynamic models that (perhaps implicitly) view the population's behaviour as stable, to dynamic ones that allow for changes in beliefs. That is, newer models allow for changes in the information set of individuals and/or experts, and even in some cases, the way that the information is interpreted. Traditional models are dynamic in the sense that there is a time-varying disease trajectory, but economic epidemiological models allow for dynamic behavioural responses. They are a function of beliefs and the ensuing actions individuals take given the constraints they face. In a traditional model the hazard of infection is an increasing function of its prevalence, but in models with behavioural dynamics the hazard rate of becoming infected might well be a decreasing function of the prevalence of the disease because of the increased demand for prevention. Beliefs interact with behaviours and affect the choices that are made, which in turn cause the information set to be updated and new beliefs to be formed. This iterative behaviour implies that much of this literature is quite mathematical and/or statistical. Some work discussed below also goes beyond population averages and looks explicitly at the heterogeneity of behavioural responses, which is an important element of the story. In the popular press, Gary Becker cites John Stuart Mill in noting the importance of adaptation in the face of natural disasters that typically leads to rapid recovery from single occurrence disasters.[1] Understanding adaptation is a central feature of economic epidemiology, and it underlies the work by James and Sargent in this volume and differentiates their analysis from the literature with more extreme findings cited in their chapter.

Dynamic behavioural response models tend to focus on individual reactions to changes in disease prevalence, but some research also addresses the interaction between those reactions and the choices/behaviours of society's institutions such as governments or various national and international agencies like the Centers for Disease Control (CDC) and the World Health Organization (WHO). Statistical modelling is common at the individual level, but not at the institutional one. Obviously, the latter is quite challenging; but it is worthwhile to think more about how alternative institutional and/or organizational forms influence infectious disease prevention and surveillance efforts. Governance issues, such as those discussed by Wilson and Lazar in this volume, appear to be increasingly important. It appears that, because of institutions' influence on individual beliefs, and because of their coordinating capacity, understanding this component may provide a large payoff for policy in the future.

Much of literature in economic epidemiology focuses on the *prevalence-elasticity* of the demand for prevention. Philipson's papers are comprehensive surveys of this topic and this section of the chapter is indebted to his work.[2] Although the details are context-specific, depending upon the nature of each disease's transmission pathology, two findings recur. First, the growth of disease is often to some extent self-limiting because an increasing prevalence causes increased private preventative behaviour. Second, at low prevalence levels, it can be difficult to eradicate an infectious disease because of the very same relationship.

Individuals Take Actions to Protect Themselves

It is not controversial to say that individuals, although sometimes altruistic, often undertake actions in accord with their own best interests, and, therefore, during an epidemic individuals take actions to protect themselves. While this observation may seem self-evident, it has not traditionally been incorporated into many statistical epidemiological models. A substantial amount of work on behavioural responses has focused on HIV/AIDS. Philipson and Posner point out that in 1988 the Centers for Disease Control predicted an accumulation of about 365,000 AIDS cases by 1992.[3] However, only about 70 percent of that number were reported in the relevant period. These authors, and others, argue that the underlying models failed to incorporate endogenous changes in behaviour. Of course, such strategic individual behaviour is more or less feasible depending upon the nature of the interaction that spreads the contagion.

In interesting and illustrative research, Dow and Philipson look at the issue of assortive matching in the transmission of HIV.[4] Most formal epidemiological modelling appears to assume that in cases where transmission requires one-on-one contact, for example the selection of sexual partners, random matching occurs. However, there is an incentive for non-infected individuals to seek out non-infected partners. Similarly, infected individuals, perhaps for altruistic and/or strategic reasons, may select infected individuals as partners. In combination, actions by both sets of parties imply that the infection rate would be less than that assumed by random matching. In the extreme, perfect assortive matching implies no transmission in the case of HIV/AIDS. Of course, an infection rate greater than that observed assuming random matching is possible if, on average, infected individuals seek out non-infected partners and/or non-infected individuals seek out infected ones. Note that assortive matching is not an assumption; rather it is an implication of the underlying assumption that individuals seek out matches that are in their own best interest.

Dow and Philipson study homosexual men in San Francisco and the HIV prevalence in the sample is roughly 50 percent. This high prevalence rate implies that the incidence of new infections is very sensitive to different levels of assortive matching. They find that HIV-positive individuals have more than twice the probability of having an HIV-positive partner than HIV-negative individuals. Of course, the observed concordant matches may be infection induced rather than incentive induced. The paper discusses this distinction and how to isolate one from the other. Overall, the incidence of new infections is implied to be reduced by between 25 and 40 percent as a result of the incentive-induced assortive matching. This implies a substantially lower rate of transmission than that observed in models of random matching. Of course, other behavioural responses also reduce the transmission rate; Gersovitz and Hammer report on the finding that discordant partners who learn of their status tend to adopt safer practices than concordant ones.[5] Understanding the range and likelihood of alternative behavioural responses is clearly an important element in understanding a disease's dynamics.

A key issue is that private infection prevention is a function of disease prevalence. Philipson points to a range of studies that observe many ramifications of this tendency.[6] For example, condom use increases with local HIV/AIDS infection rates; flu shots are most likely to be taken up by those at greatest risk of infection; and the vaccination rate for measles, mumps, and rubella (MMR) varies with the local caseload. For public policy purposes, understanding this prevalence-elastic behaviour is an element of effective program design.

Auld extends this earlier work and estimates dynamic models of behavioural responses to the HIV/AIDS epidemic with a focus on individual choices and beliefs.[7] His statistical modelling suggests some perhaps counterintuitive outcomes are possible. In particular, when individuals hold pessimistic expectations about the future time path of the epidemic's prevalence they are more likely to engage in risky behaviour. Moreover, individuals' beliefs about the probability that they are already infected can influence their actions markedly. Behavioural responses can cause the disease to spread more or less quickly. He observes that information can affect the time path of the incidence of the prevalence of the infection. A policy intervention, for example a preventive vaccine, can have quite different impacts depending on whether it is anticipated or not. Individuals who anticipated a cure or vaccine are more likely to increase their risk-taking behaviour. He also quantifies how individuals adjust their risky behaviour in response to disease prevalence for HIV/AIDS. On average, risky behaviour is reduced by 5 percent in response to a 10 percent increase in disease prevalence. However, there is substantial heterogeneity across individuals. Low-risk individuals reduce risky behaviour substantially more than high-risk ones. This heterogeneity implies significant challenges for public policy.

Underlying both Dow and Philipson's and Auld's work are assumptions about the utility that is gained from establishing a match, or pursuing risky behaviours more generally, as well as the information that individuals are able to ascertain about a potential match's infection status. Information is crucial and diagnostic testing, a key means of reducing uncertainty and improving information, can have very different implications across different subgroups of the population. Some, such as Philipson and Posner, even argue that it can lead to increased incidence in some environments.[8] Gersovitz and Hammer discuss this in the context of a population comprising altruists and egoists.[9] Surveying the international literature, they report the common finding that many of those tested do not return for their results. One study finds that a significant percentage of those who test HIV-positive do not tell their partners.

In the case of SARS, there were many newspaper accounts of individuals taking, whether well or poorly informed, preventative measures in an effort to both avoid infecting others and becoming infected.[10] Diverse actions included wearing masks in public, or at least while on public transit or in other situations involving close human contact, and accepting voluntary quarantine. In Toronto, upon hearing in the media of a putative relationship between the infection and the Chinese community, many stopped going to Chinese restaurants. Gersovitz and Hammer point to the common practice in Japan of individuals attempting to limit their likelihood of infecting others by wearing face masks when they have the common cold or flu virus.[11] Grace Wong analyzes the impact of SARS on the Hong Kong property market as a result of individual actions to avoid high-prevalence areas.[12]

Societies and Investors Take Actions to Protect Themselves

Although much less formally studied in the contemporary economic epidemiology literature, the role of government and other institutions during an outbreak or a potential outbreak usually has substantial economic impacts. Moreover, and this appears to be of increasing importance, the economic ramifications of what would be considered relatively small outbreaks by historical norms, or even the threat of an outbreak, can be very substantial because of the magnifying effect of actions by government and related agencies/organizations. Of course, while such action is costly, it also (hopefully) has a substantial preventative effect. Further, as society becomes wealthier it is willing (even desires) to purchase greater insurance against major calamities and this type of strong action can be seen as a form of insurance. The large-scale destruction of animals in the face of not only major, but more minor, indications of disease is an example of such behaviour. Recent examples include reactions to bovine spongiform encephalopathy (BSE) in cattle, and the avian flu in fowl. See the WHO's information pages for details of both of these.[13] The problem is that action by one government can be sub-optimal (either too large or small depending upon the context) since it does not fully take into account the costs and benefits it is imposing on other jurisdictions, and government action can have substantial consequences.

Governments can, however, influence and coordinate private activities to great effect. For example, in an important public relations and information dissemination exercise the Canadian prime minister and a number of his staff ate lunch in a Chinese restaurant in Toronto as a tangible indication that eating in Asian restaurants in Toronto was safe.[14] In addition to public health authorities quarantining many high-risk individuals, a large number not quarantined imposed on themselves a sort of quasi-quarantine by restricting their interaction with groups and individuals whom they perceived to be high-risk. Of course, some of these actions have costs that the individual decisionmaker does not fully recognize and/or take into account. In the social context, Janet Davies of the Canadian Nurses Association reports that the children of health-care workers were ostracized during the SARS crisis due to the perceived threat from their parents' occupation.[15] Overall, the effectiveness of the self-motivated preventative actions in the SARS crisis remains unclear; however, the scale of the private response is appreciable and can be more so if coordinated by, for example, WHO travel advisories.[16] Providing appropriate and credible information in order to motivate appropriate infection transmission-reduction behaviour can have a very real impact on the time path of the prevalence of the infection. In the absence of information, people tend to be risk-averse and follow a precautionary principle in their private behaviours. In the face of substantial uncertainty, especially when the transmission mechanism is not fully understood, governments, and domestic and international organizations such as the WHO, walk a tightrope between encouraging or channelling private prevention and minimizing the economic impact of those same preventative behaviours, for example, in the area of tourism. These two motivations can be (and frequently are) at odds with each other. Designing appropriate institutional structures to generate and analyze appropriate data on all sides of the issue(s), inform and make appropriate decisions, and communicate in a clear and non-contradictory manner, is crucial to the well-being of society. The design phase, of course, needs to be accomplished well before a crisis takes hold, and one such design issue is discussed by Wilson and Lazar in this volume. Note that aggregate business activity tends to be somewhat less affected by short duration crises, although specific sectors and/or locations can have substantial negative (e.g., Toronto's Asian restaurants) or positive (e.g., those who sell transmission-reducing supplies) experiences.

The basic idea that individuals manage risk during an epidemic, balancing perceived probabilities of infection with the expected gains of pursuing, or losses from not pursing, costly activities may seem straightforward, but formally modelling it so as to have a better information base for prediction in future occurrences remains a challenge. Understanding and predicting individual actions is important since government can substantially alter the costs of individual actions. For example, during the SARS outbreak in Canada the federal government increased the generosity of the Employment Insurance (called Unemployment Insurance in many countries) system for those accepting voluntary quarantine, thereby reducing compliance costs and making acceptance much more likely. Job losses were, of course, also prevented by legislation requiring firms to preserve jobs for quarantined workers. Still, compliance was an issue during the outbreak, as it is in many similar situations. This points out the importance of institutional responses and the incentives they create, which interact with individual behaviour. In this case, my view is that government compensation from this and other sources was neither as early, widely publicized, nor as substantial as would have been warranted if it was believed that selected quarantine was really a desirable and effective measure.

Criticisms are sometimes made regarding government reactions to epidemics. For example, Philipson points out that many US states have been criticized for their slowness in instituting HIV/AIDS prevention programs.[17] However, economic epidemiology suggests that much policy is driven by (local) prevalence, not calendar time (although it may be the expectation of the prevalence that matters). When access to prevention programs is viewed through a prevalence lens, the public sector's response seems more plausible since high-prevalence states acted more rapidly while low-prevalence states employed their resources for other purposes, although their timelines may not be criticism-free. A related interesting issue is that as the prevalence of a disease increases (at least for common pathologies) the marginal value of the public programs tends to decrease since many individuals are already taking protective action privately.[18] This implies that the larger the existing caseload, the smaller the incremental value of government programs. It follows that the optimal timing of many government interventions is early, when they can have a larger effect for the cost. Also, this perspective speaks to the alternative mechanisms that governments employ in fighting an infection, which can be broadly classified as subsidization (or incentives) and regulation (or mandating). After initial efforts to fight an epidemic have been undertaken, subsidization may become prohibitively expensive since those who face the lowest cost of taking preventative action have already done so. Therefore, mandating compliance may become socially beneficial. Boozer and Philipson find evidence of behaviour consistent with regulation dominating subsidization for HIV/AIDS programs in some contexts.[19]

The externalities associated with the international transmission of diseases are more complex than in the past given increasing globalization, and many costs are imposed by one country on another without being fully internalized by the country making the decision.[20] Although national actions are part of the give and take of international diplomacy and trade, reactions to epidemics are not treated/viewed the same way as most other trade or diplomatic skirmishes and very high costs can be imposed by one country on another. This is particularly the case when there are new diseases/infections where there is a great deal of uncertainty. The international transmission of health information regarding outbreaks has long been an element (although perhaps not always a front-page element) of international diplomacy. Bell and Lewis point out that the 1918 influenza epidemic served to strengthen the health aspects of the League of Nations in subsequent years, and recent government actions (and inactions) around SARS are affecting the WHO's charter and international information-gathering strategy.[21]

The type of international externality described is difficult to address and is in the ambit of international diplomacy. Examples of such actions include several recent cases of closing international borders to beef imports as a result of sometimes substantial, but sometimes isolated, positive tests for the so-called mad cow disease and various strains of avian influenza. Another is not providing complete or timely information about contagions that are occurring in one jurisdiction so that others can take preventative action. This class of issue also includes travel advisories issued by the WHO during the SARS outbreak. Bell and Lewis point out that at the peak of the SARS crisis almost half of flights to Southeast Asia were cancelled and passenger arrivals declined by two-thirds.[22]

Bell and Lewis also emphasize the importance of expectations and psychological sentiment in driving policy decisions, with errors in both directions, especially before the scale and nature of an outbreak are clear. Expectations with large economic implications also operate through the interaction of public and quasi-public institutions with private ones. The massive drop in, for example, Eurobond spreads in China at the onset of the SARS crisis is a case in point indicating a drop in business confidence. Alsan, Bloom and Canning investigate how foreign direct investment responds to health status, noting that for China it fell by US$2.7 billion during the SARS crisis, and by 62 percent for one quarter in Hong Kong in the same year.[23] However, these drops reversed as quickly as did the crisis once the limited nature of the syndrome was understood. Longer-term domestic health status (proxied by life expectancy) is found to be one of the most quantifiably important determinants of foreign direct investment controlling for a range of other relevant factors. Longer lasting epidemics, such as HIV/AIDS or malaria can have severe impacts on the capital structure, and thereby the productivity and standard of living of a country. David Francis emphasizes that poor health and high infectious disease rates have a direct effect on workers and their output, and an indirect effect on worker productivity through reduced physical capital formation.[24]

THE COST OF INFECTION

Basic program evaluation or cost-benefit analysis usually defines three types of costs (and benefits): direct, such as hospital or nursing services; indirect, such as a loss of tourism dollars; and, intangible, such as the loss of pleasure from tourist activities. Many traditional cost-of-illness analyses, such as those by the WHO and CDC, appear to focus primarily on the direct costs of morbidity and mortality.[25] Recently, especially in the case of SARS, there has been a greater recognition of the indirect costs. Some infection-avoidance programs primarily induce indirect costs and these can be substantial. Further, Philipson argues that the intangible costs can be much more important than has been appreciated and can justify substantial expenditures on prevention as well as research and development.[26]

Governments, international agencies, and the like operate in a world of risk management, and expected crises do not always materialize, or do not do so at the time or in the manner expected. A classic example, documented by Neustadt and Fineberg, concerns the anticipated swine flu epidemic in 1976 in the United States.[27] Not only did the influenza outbreak not materialize, but the vaccination program had serious side effects for a small fraction of the treated population. Discussing risk management for what is commonly known as undulant fever, O'Riordan analyzed the costs and benefits of preventing a ban on cattle imports to the United States.[28] The risk never materialized, though a similar cattle-related event is underway now, but he clearly demonstrated the considerable economic harm of such a closure and points out the substantial prevention program warranted by even the risk of enduring the economic impact of a border closure.

PUBLIC DECISION-MAKING ABOUT PUBLIC HEALTH AND INFECTIOUS DISEASE CONTROL

Both directly and through arm's-length agencies, governments are the key institutions that serve to provide preventative programs, disease surveillance, and other public health services. But, they also provide and regulate a wide range of completely unrelated areas and have scarce resources that they shift across dramatically different priorities. Therefore, they must make trade-offs and choices in the face of voter opinion and many other constraints. Economic theory suggests that what optimizing governments, in fact all decisionmakers, will do is to equalize the ratio of the present discounted value of the marginal benefit of each activity relative to that activity's price across all endeavours.[29]

Of course, in the political context that is government decision-making, the price includes more than financial costs. A shorthand version of the principle suggests that (assuming the prices of alternatives are the same for illustrative simplicity) if the marginal benefit of an activity is greater than that of the alternatives, then the resources available to it should be increased. As a particular activity is pursued, implying it has a high marginal benefit, its marginal benefit will decline until some other activity has a higher one and resources are shifted to that new alternative. While such a strategy can never be perfectly accomplished given that information is limited (it is especially difficult to measure benefits and prices in this context since they include many intangible and/or political factors) and the prices and marginal value of benefits are constantly shifting, it is nevertheless a useful guide with predictive power. Resources are taken away from activities where their removal will cause the least harm and allocated to activities where they will have the greatest benefit (or, relative benefit if prices vary across activities).

One relevant observation that follows from equalizing marginal benefit to price ratios is that most infections will not be completely eliminated. Assume for simplicity that prices are fixed; as an infection's prevalence declines, the marginal benefit of fighting it also declines and soon the marginal benefit of some other activity will become relatively larger. Resources will soon be shifted to that next best alternative. One, sometimes more than theoretical, exception to this is that governments and similar organizations may solve an externality and recognize a greater benefit than do private individuals. Many of the beneficiaries of eradication are children and future generations, who cannot bear current costs for an eradication program. Hence, there is an intergenerational externality that can motivate government action to eradicate the disease through debt financing. Of course, there are other times when eradication will be pursued, such as, for example, when there is a high probability of there being a near-term resurgence that would have great costs.

One implication of equating marginal benefit to price ratios across alternatives — that is, balancing the great diversity of needs and wants of society and allocating resources to where they get "the biggest bang for their buck" — is that, whether conscious or implicit, governments trade off public health and infection control for other benefits. Substantial public funds in both Canada and the United States are spent, for example, on television programming and various cultural events that could be diverted to health care.[30] That the funds are not allocated to health points to the great value that society places on these other activities. Governments seek the "greater good," which sometimes implies, as revealed by government actions, spending money in promoting popular culture instead of public health.

A clear example of balancing unrelated costs and benefits, not involving infectious diseases but public health more broadly, is the Canadian and US experience with highway speeds. The economic issues and mortality trade-offs of the US experience have been documented by Orley Ashenfelter and Michael Greenstone.[31] Following the oil shocks of the mid-1970s, speed limits were reduced on interstate freeways by the US federal government to conserve fuel. A number of studies were completed by the 1980s that clearly, consistently, and convincingly showed the causal relationship between higher highway speed limits and increased mortality (and other negative effects of highway motor vehicle accidents). Nevertheless, reduced speeds are costly in the sense that they increase travel times. Hence, in 1987 the US federal government allowed state governments to raise rural interstate speed limits. Most, but not all, states increased their speed limits over time and some increased their limits more than others. Some Canadian provinces, such as New Brunswick and Alberta, have also elected to have higher speed limits. As Ashenfelter and Greenstone show, the legislators clearly understood that they were making a trade-off between mortality (and morbidity) and reduced travel times — and most elected reduced travel times.

As can be seen in the previous example, public health and by extension programs related to epidemics are constantly being compared to, and quite explicitly traded-off against, other priorities of society. During the SARS crisis there was much debate about economic costs compared to the medical efficacy of travel advisories and quarantine. In terms of government and policy, political decisions made around the Cabinet table always trade off such factors.[32] Funds are regularly allocated between, for example, public health and other government activities such as, in the Canadian context, the Canadian

Broadcasting Corporation (CBC – federally) or TV Ontario (TVO – provincially). While normally implicit, comparisons between factors, including mortality, that are not obviously comparable are regularly compared nevertheless, and decisions are made to allocate resources to one or another. Implicitly or explicitly, and sometimes quite inconsistently from one issue or jurisdiction to the next, people make judgements about the value of human lives.

HETEROGENEITY

Heterogeneity in tastes and demands for service raise a serious dilemma in the debate about public versus private funding, and public and private action, in infectious disease prevention and control (and also in health care more generally). This debate is particularly vociferous in jurisdictions such as Canada with nationalized health-care systems, but is equally true in the US where public health is effectively nationalized (or at least government run). While this is an oversimplification, at its essence the problem is that governments must choose a single level of funding, and a single level of service quality, for a jurisdiction.[33] A common criterion discussed in the medical literature is about $50,000 per quality-adjusted life-year (QALY).[34] In contrast to this relative homogeneity, individual valuations of personal health and tastes for health-related risk vary markedly and individuals are prepared to expend dramatically different levels of resources on their own, and their family's, health care. Part of this follows from different levels of income/wealth, but much variation occurs for those of comparable income levels. Whatever single level of service a government chooses, there will be some who view it as too little and others who view it as too much (holding prices constant); or, at least, there will be some who want to put more resources to that end, while others desire to allocate fewer. Public policy walks a tight rope between the alternative demands of a diverse society.

CONCLUSION

Many of the key ideas of economic epidemiology are centred on the concept of the prevalence-elastic behaviour of the population — the private demand for prevention varies with the prevalence rate. This includes the dynamic feedback of information affecting beliefs and then actions, which in turn affect the time-path of disease prevalence. This can be clearly seen in the case of SARS where individuals undertook a variety of measures that were expected to be self-protective. Public policy plays an important role in informing beliefs and conditioning actions. Further, government and international organizations can magnify and/or coordinate, for better or worse, private infection-avoidance behaviours. These behaviours can, of course, have very substantial economic implications, especially when coordinated, and some perhaps unexpected implications flow from this model's view of the world; for example, subjective self-assessments of the probability of already being infected can have substantial impacts on behaviour and disease transmission.

Government action in the face of a crisis, or the expectation of one, also plays a crucial role in aligning private actions. Moreover, increasing globalization implies that different governments can impose benefits and/or costs on each other's jurisdictions without fully internalizing the benefits and costs of doing so.

It is also useful to consider the challenges faced in government, or societal, decision-making. Governments allocate resources across an incredibly wide range of areas, and trade off, frequently implicitly, mortality against alternative resource allocations that many think of as philosophically incomparable. The context and heterogeneity in society is such that it is virtually impossible to satisfy all members with a single decision. Nevertheless, a single decision is often called for. There is still much to be learned about the interrelationships between private behaviour and tastes, and public institutional structures. In fact, it is probably an area of research that will have a large payoff for public health and infectious disease-control.

NOTES

[1]Gary S. Becker "... And the Economics of Disaster Management," *The Wall Street Journal* (New York), 4 January 2005, p. A12.

[2]T. Philipson, "Economic Epidemiology and Public Health," in *New Economics of Human Behavior: Essays in Honor of Gary Becker*, ed. M. Tommasi and K. Ierulli (Cambridge: Cambridge University Press, 1995), pp. 216-35, and "Economic Epidemiology and Infectious Disease," in *Handbook of Health Economics*, ed. J. Newhouse and T. Culyer (New York: North-Holland, 2000). For a brief and more general overview of relevant issues in health economics, see C. Auld, C. Donaldson, C. Mitton and P. Shackley, "Health Economics," in *Oxford Textbook of Public Health* (4th edition), ed. R. Detels, J. McEwen, R. Beaglehole and H.T. Tamaka (Oxford: Oxford University Press, 2001).

[3]T. Philipson and R.A. Posner, *Private Choices and Public Health: An Economic Interpretation of the AIDS Epidemic* (Cambridge, MA: Harvard University Press, 1993).

[4]W.H. Dow and T. Philipson, "An Empirical Examination of Assortative Matching on the Incidence of HIV," *Journal of Health Economics* 15, no. 6 (1996):735-52, and "Assortative Matching and the Growth of Infectious Disease," *Mathematical Biosciences* 148, no. 2 (1998):161-81.

[5]Mark Gersovitz and Jeffrey S. Hammer, "Infectious Diseases, Public Policy, and the Marriage of Economics and Epidemiology," *The World Bank Research Observer* 18, no. 2 (2003):129-57.

[6]Philipson, "Economic Epidemiology and Infectious Disease."

[7]M.C. Auld, "Choices, Beliefs, and Infectious Disease Dynamics," *Journal of Health Economics* 22, no. 3 (2003):361-77, and "Estimating Behavioral Response to the AIDS Epidemic," *Contributions to Economic Analysis and Policy* 5, no. 1 (2006): Article 12. At www.bepress.com/bejeap/contributions/vol5/iss1/art12.

[8]Philipson and Posner, *Private Choices and Public Health,* p. 84.

[9]Gersovitz and Hammer, "Infectious Diseases, Public Policy, and the Marriage of Economics and Epidemiology."

[10]For discussions of the SARS crisis, see Independent SARS Commission (Mr. Justice Archie Campbell, chair), *SARS and Public Health Legislation,* Second Interim Report (Toronto: The Commission, 2005), pp. 423 plus appendices, at www.sarscommission.ca/; Alexis Lau, "The Numbers Trail: What the Data Tells Us," in *At the Epicentre: Hong Kong and the SARS Outbreak,* ed. Christine Loh and Civic Exchange (Aberdeen, Hong Kong: Hong Kong University Press, 2004), pp. 81-94; and Stephen Brown, "The Economic Impact of SARS," in *At the Epicentre: Hong Kong and the SARS Outbreak,* pp. 179-93.

[11]Gersovitz and Hammer, "Infectious Diseases, Public Policy, and the Marriage of Economics and Epidemiology."

[12]Grace Wong, "Has SARS Infected the Property Market? Evidence from Hong Kong," Working Paper no. 488 (Princeton, NJ: Industrial Relations Section, Princeton University, 2004).

[13]World Health Organization, "Avian Flu Web information page" at www.who.int/csr/disease/avian_influenza/en/index.html, and the "Bovine spongiform encephalopathy (BSE) page" at www.who.int/zoonoses/diseases/bse/en/.

[14]Canadian Press wire service, "Chrétien Aims to Dispel SARS Fears," 10 April 2003.

[15]Reported in Thomas S. Axworthy, "An Ounce of Prevention," in *The National Post,* 19 May 2006, p. A12. Article was based on a presentation at a Queen's University School of Policy Studies conference on disaster management.

[16]The impact of the SARS-associated reduction in travel on the tourism industry, and direct costs to workers as a result of SARS, were addressed for Toronto and Ontario by provincial legislation — the *SARS Assistance and Recovery Strategy Act,* 2003. An independent commission was set up to investigate SARS in Ontario. The

Campbell Commission reports on many of the financial issues for Ontario. See the Second Interim Report of the Independent SARS Commission.

[17]Philipson, "Economic Epidemiology and Infectious Disease," section 3.3.

[18]For an expansion of this analysis, which is motivated primarily by HIV/AIDS, see P. Geoffard and T. Philipson, "Rational Epidemics and their Public Control," *International Economic Review* 37, no. 3 (1996):603-24, and "Disease Eradication: Public vs. Private Vaccination," *American Economic Review* 87, no. 1 (1997):221-31.

[19]M. Boozer and T. Philipson, "The Impact of Public Testing for Human Immunodeficiency Virus," *Journal of Human Resources* 35, no. 3 (2000):419-46.

[20]Of course, many if not all of international trade-related responses should be interpreted as having multiple motivations. While there may be substantial costs to some sectors following from, for example, an import ban, other sectors may gain appreciably.

[21]C. Bell and Maureen Lewis, "The Economic Implications of Epidemics Old and New," Working Paper No. 54 (Washington, DC: Center for Global Development, 2005). For more information on the WHO and SARS, see the WHO's "Web information page" at www.who.int/csr/sars/en.

[22]Bell and Lewis, "The Economic Implications of Epidemics Old and New."

[23]Marcella Alsan, David E. Bloom and David Canning, "The Effect of Population Health on Foreign Direct Investment," NBER Working Paper No. 10596 (Cambridge, MA: National Bureau of Economic Research, 2004). At www.nber.org.

[24]David R. Francis, "Better Health Increases Foreign Direct Investment," *NBER Digest* (2005):4.

[25]Of course, these analyses either implicitly or explicitly choose some monetary value for a life. A wide range of valuations is possible and this choice is quite important to the final magnitude obtained in each study.

[26]Philipson, "Economic Epidemiology and Infectious Disease."

[27]Richard E. Neustadt and Harvey Fineberg, *The Epidemic that Never Was: Policy-Making and the Swine Flu Affair* (New York: Vintage Books, 1983; 1st edition 1982).

[28]Fred O'Riordan, "An Economic Evaluation of Alternative Programs to Control Brucellosis in Canadian Cattle," *Canadian Farm Economics* 15 (June):1-26.

[29]There is some informal debate between those who believe that (at least academic) economics should be primarily or exclusively descriptive, and those who think that it should be proscriptive. It appears to be a bit of each. A marginal benefit is defined as the value derived from a small increase in the output level of an activity. Although only increases are mentioned for simplicity, the concept applies equally to decreases.

[30]I point to cultural industries to emphasize the range of activities of government. The issue applies equally well to expenditure on other categories of consumption.

[31]Orley Ashenfelter and Michael Greenstone, "Estimating the Value of a Statistical Life: The Importance of Omitted Variables and Publication Bias," *American Economic Review* 94, no. 2 (May 2004):454-60, and "Using Mandated Speed Limits

to Measure the Value of a Statistical Life," *Journal of Political Economy* 112, no. S1 (February 2004):226-67.

[32]Although not the focus of this example, individuals also regularly make trade-offs between health and activities/items that appear to be completely unrelated, and their choices commonly affect others.

[33]It is clear that this statement is too strong. There are, for example, different levels of service in rural compared to urban areas. But, this does not take away from the main idea, which is that the level of service is quite homogeneous.

[34]A. Laupacis, "Inclusion of Drugs in Provincial Drug Benefit Programs: Who Is Making these Decisions, and Are they the Right Ones?" [editorial], *Canadian Medical Association Journal* 166, no. 1 (2002):44-47. A. Laupacis, D. Feeny, A.S. Detsky and P.X. Tugwell, "How Attractive Does a New Technology Have to be to Warrant Adoption and Utilization? Tentative Guidelines for Using Clinical and Economic Evaluations," *Canadian Medical Association Journal* 146 (1992):473-81.

10

GOVERNANCE IN PANDEMICS: DEFINING THE FEDERAL GOVERNMENT'S ROLE IN PUBLIC HEALTH EMERGENCIES

Kumanan Wilson and Harvey Lazar

INTRODUCTION

Public health renewal has emerged as an important policy issue in Canada, largely in response to the outbreak of SARS in Toronto in 2003 and in preparation for a possible avian flu pandemic. Of particular concern has been the capacity of this country to respond to public health emergencies in a rapid, coordinated, and effective manner. In attempting to address this issue, the federal government has chosen to take a largely collaborative approach with the provinces, on the assumption that effective relations between orders of government can be maintained in the event of an emergency.[1] In doing so, Ottawa is choosing not to adopt new legislation that could provide the federal government with the additional authority that might be needed in the event that intergovernmental relations turn out to be otherwise insufficiently effective during a crisis.

This chapter will explore some of the policy options available to the federal government when considering its role in responding to public health emergencies. An integral part of the public health renewal process will be to better define federal jurisdiction and responsibilities in the event of a public health emergency. At present there remains some uncertainty in this regard, the consequences of which could be considerable in the event of a major new

This chapter is a revised version of "Planning for the Next Pandemic Threat: Defining the Federal Role in Public Health Emergencies," *Policy Matters* 6, no. 5 (2005):1-36. At www.irpp.org/pm/archive/pmvol6no5.pdf. Reproduced with permission of the Institute for Research on Public Policy, Montreal, Quebec.

infectious threat. This chapter argues that a redefinition of federal capacity to respond to public health emergencies must be a priority of the current legislative renewal process. We believe that amendments to the current *Emergencies Act* — or the creation of new separate emergency public health legislation — that take into consideration unique aspects of public health emergencies should be a top priority in this country's efforts to ready itself to respond to the threat of a pandemic.

FEDERAL POWER IN PUBLIC HEALTH

A variety of recent threats have focused Canadian policymakers' attention on the health protection and disease prevention components of public health as they relate to infectious disease in particular. These include the discovery of bovine spongiform encephalopathy (BSE or mad cow disease), the emergence of West Nile virus, the threat of bio-terrorism and the impact of SARS. Canada's response to the outbreak of SARS clearly demonstrated the crucial need for effective governance to manage an outbreak, while exposing some of the limitations of the governance structures that existed at the time. The details of the management of the outbreak have been well described in several reports.[2] To summarize, SARS was originally identified as a case of atypical pneumonia in Guangdong Province in China in November 2002. In February 2003, the first Canadian case arrived in Toronto, sparking an outbreak that eventually affected 438 individuals and resulted in 44 deaths. The outbreak also had a negative impact on the economy of Toronto, partly due to an advisory issued by the World Health Organization (WHO) recommending against travel to the city.[3] Managing the spread of SARS presented a considerable challenge to all orders of government, largely because of a lack of knowledge about several critical aspects of the pathogen, including its level of infectivity and the exact mode of transmission.[4] In Toronto, the initial management of the outbreak occurred at the hospital and local public health levels in the areas where the disease first appeared. The provincial government soon became involved and declared the situation an emergency, allowing the government to employ aggressive protective measures such as quarantine.[5] Among the federal government's responsibilities in the management of SARS was providing epidemiologic and laboratory support to provincial and local officials; managing issues related to the spread of the disease at international borders; and communicating information on the status of the outbreak to other provinces, international organizations, and other nations.[6]

Limits on Federal Power

When considering mechanisms by which the federal government could have involved itself to a greater extent in Ontario, it soon becomes apparent that there are real limitations on Ottawa's power to act unless it has the consent of the affected province. The federal government's ability to act in a public health emergency is largely governed by two pieces of legislation: the *Emergencies Act*[7] and the *Emergency Preparedness Act*.[8] The *Emergency Preparedness Act* primarily serves as companion legislation to the *Emergencies Act*, and provides authority for the provinces and federal government to act collaboratively to prepare for an emergency. On the other hand, the *Emergencies Act*, which replaced the federal *War Measures Act* in 1985, provides the federal government with authority to take action to address a "national emergency." Under this act an infectious outbreak (disease in human beings, animals or plants) is one of several categories of emergency considered to be a "public welfare emergency." Others include accidents, pollution, and natural disasters. The *Emergencies Act* confers substantial powers on the federal government to control public welfare emergencies. These include the regulation of travel to the affected region, evacuation of the area, possession of property, and the direction of services to provide emergency care. In general, these would be considered adequate powers to manage an infectious outbreak. However, the act also provides an important limit on federal power, by specifically stating that:

> The Governor in Council may not issue a declaration of a public welfare emergency where the direct effects of the emergency are confined to, or occur principally in, one province unless the lieutenant governor in council of the province has indicated to the Governor in Council that the emergency exceeds the capacity or authority of the province to deal with it.[9]

It appears that the single province constraint in the existing emergency legislation has more applicability to accidents and natural disasters, which by their nature are likely to be confined to a single geographic area. It is much less obvious that the federal government should be similarly constrained in the case of an infectious disease outbreak. According to the existing legislation, the federal government must ask permission before being allowed to take action to control a disease outbreak that has occurred in only one province. The implications of this limitation to federal powers were evident in the management of SARS, which in Canada was primarily confined to Ontario, although it was present in 26 other countries.[10] By not having the necessary authority, the federal government was dependent on provincial cooperation for information on the nature and extent of the outbreak. It soon became evident that cooperation between the provincial and federal governments was less than optimal. This was well documented by the Campbell report, which examined the management of the outbreak in Ontario.[11] The report, in particular, identified the dysfunctional relationship between the provincial chief medical officer and federal officials. The poor relationship had several consequences, including inadequate data transfer to the federal level and the recall of federal field epidemiologists from Ontario due to lack of clarity about their role. The problems with intergovernmental cooperation were noted not only in Canada but also by international agencies. David Heymann of the WHO commented that:

> SARS has shown us that relationships between federal, or central, and provincial or state governments are very important in public health, and very difficult to establish.... We understand that this has been a problem in China. It certainly has been a problem in Canada, where there have been difficulties between Health Canada and the provincial government.[12]

Concerns over the existing emergency legislation and the limitations on federal power were highlighted in the reports by Dr. Naylor and Senator Kirby.[13] Advocating legislative renewal as a possible solution, the Canadian Medical Association (CMA) has proposed a *Canadian Emergency Health Measures Act* based on a health-alert system. This proposal outlines five levels of health alert. For each level it describes associated governmental powers, whether consent of the province is required for action and who the lead response team would be. The CMA proposal also suggests that the share of federal funding of the crisis should progressively increase as the level of alert increases.[14] The Naylor report supported this approach and in particular highlighted the importance of having a graded system.[15] The Kirby report echoed these sentiments and endorsed a mildly modified version of the CMA system. While several of the recommendations of both the Naylor and Kirby reports have been implemented, little progress has been made in relation to their recommendations regarding the need for new emergency legislation.

CONCERNS WITH EXISTING INTERGOVERNMENTAL RELATIONSHIPS

National Concerns

Many of the current reform initiatives have attempted to address these dysfunctional relationships, primarily by developing better communication strategies and intergovernmental interfaces. Under the previous Liberal government, Ottawa has moved on two broad fronts to improve its capacity on public health emergency preparedness and response. The first front was the federal strategy on public health. Led by the minister of health and the minister of state for public health, this strategy has been composed of three key elements: the creation of the Public Health Agency of Canada (PHAC), the appointment of a chief public health officer for Canada and the development of the Pan-Canadian Public Health Network. The second front of the federal response has been contained in the government's national security framework and action plan, *Securing an Open Society: Canada's National Security Policy.*[16] This framework seeks to build a fully-integrated security system that brings together, and provides tools to better coordinate, the federal government's security capacity. The national security framework aims at integrating efforts to renew the federal government's leadership in public health with its broader action plan for emergency preparedness.

Despite these initiatives, there remain shortcomings with the current set of intergovernmental arrangements, which depend upon the voluntary cooperation of provinces at the time of a public health crisis. Fundamentally, the issues relate to externalities and spillovers of disease outbreaks. A disease developing in one province affects not only that one province; it has the potential to affect other provinces across the country, either directly through spread of the disease or indirectly through stigmatization of the affected region. Thus, in many respects, the management of a disease outbreak is of national concern. If a province has the resources to adequately manage the outbreak, there would be no requirement for assistance from the federal government. However, at a minimum, a province should communicate information on the outbreak openly to other governments. Such information would allow adjacent provinces to prepare for the potential spread of the disease. Unfortunately, there may also be disincentives for a provincial government to provide detailed reporting of the status of an outbreak in its territory, particularly at an early stage when there is uncertainty about the outbreak's magnitude and when such reporting could, perhaps unnecessarily, adversely affect that province's industries and tourism. Thus, it is conceivable that a province would be reluctant to report an outbreak out of fear of negative economic consequences or simply out of a belief that the matter was within its sole jurisdiction. This would be particularly worrisome if that province proved not to be able to manage the outbreak effectively on its own and had not provided adequate reporting to other governments. Apart from the health impacts of the spread of the disease across the country, there would also be concerns about the potential for stigmatization, which would likely not be confined to the province initially affected, particularly if international attention were drawn to the outbreak. Similarly, if an outbreak involved a specific industry within the affected province, and international attention were drawn to the matter, that industry could be affected nationwide. The federal government might also have a disincentive to report on the status of an outbreak, but since its electoral accountability is to the entire country, rather than only to the region where the outbreak would be occurring, the disincentive to report is comparatively less than that experienced by a single province.

A vivid illustration of the importance of a national approach to combating a developing outbreak is provided by two simulations of a human-to-human avian flu outbreak developing in Southeast Asia.[17] While varying in their estimation of the potential severity of the outbreak, both simulations do suggest that the outbreak could be stopped with aggressive early interventions. These interventions would include pre-pandemic flu vaccination, social distancing measures such as quarantine and the targeted distribution of antiviral treatments. While an emerging human avian flu pandemic in Canada would have different characteristics, the fundamental principles of the response to the outbreak would likely apply in this country as well. Early detection of the outbreak and the mobilization of adequate public health resources to introduce preventative measures would be necessary to halt the epidemic. Such an operation would likely require a national effort with public health resources from the entire country being diverted to the affected province. Ideally, this would be a collaborative enterprise between the Public Health Agency of Canada and provincial and local public officials. However, if for some of the reasons described above a province were slow to report the outbreak or hesitant to allow federal involvement, an otherwise preventable epidemic might spread to adjacent provinces. While federal intervention would by then be statutorily permissible, the window of opportunity for effective action would have passed.

International Concerns

The recent emergence of a new international approach to combat pandemic infections adds to the urgency of addressing Canadian governance strategies related to the management of infectious outbreaks at a national level. This new model of global health governance has developed principally in response to SARS. A key component of this more aggressive approach to the management of pandemics concerns the responsibility of individual nations to the global community with regard to adequate national surveillance and communication of the status of outbreaks to the WHO. Canada's roles and responsibilities as part of the larger international community provide compelling reasons for a re-evaluation of the current federal approach to public health emergencies.

In many ways the international health community could be viewed historically as a confederation, with the WHO acting on behalf of member states of the World Health Assembly. In this model, the WHO was necessarily subordinate to the member nations, in accordance with the principle of the primacy of national sovereignty. But this model is being replaced. As well described by David Fidler, Lawrence Gostin and others, a transformation in governance regime is occurring.[18] Now, in times of disease outbreaks, the WHO can act in many ways as a central authority with considerable coercive power over its member states. In Fidler's language, global germ governance is being, or perhaps already has been, transformed from a horizontal governance regime to one that is more characterized by a vertical relationship.[19] In the horizontal governance regime the objective of the International Health Regulations, the primary piece of legislation governing the international management of disease outbreaks, was to prevent the spread of disease from nation to nation with minimal interruption of international traffic or trade. In this governance regime the sovereignty of individual nations was paramount, and the WHO did not have the authority to act in a nation without its permission. In the transition to a vertical governance regime, however, the WHO has begun to act directly within nations to control the spread of disease. The management of SARS demonstrated how aggressive this governance regime could be, largely as a consequence of two new approaches the WHO has adopted. The WHO has received authority from the World Health Assembly to use non-governmental sources of information to track the spread of disease.[20] An application of this authority is the use of information provided by the Global Public Health Intelligence Network (GPHIN). GPHIN was developed by Health Canada and is employed by the WHO to scour international Web sites for evidence of disease outbreaks.[21] The ability to use non-governmental sources of information is significant because it allows the WHO to conduct surveillance without member nation permission. The second component of what Fidler describes as the WHO's "double-pincer" power over nations is its ability to issue travel advisories.[22] Though they were not explicitly authorized, travel advisories were used by the WHO in combating SARS.[23] And while there was some disagreement with the decision to issue travel advisories based on scientific grounds, the right of the WHO to issue such advisories appears not to have been questioned. The ability to conduct independent surveillance and to make unilateral declarations of travel advisories provides the WHO with considerable power to govern the international management of an outbreak. Specifically, attempts by countries to withhold information will likely ultimately fail — due to the acquisition of information from non-governmental sources — and result in penalties in the form of travel advisories.

This changing state of international governance has important implications for Canada. Our federal government must have the ability to acquire complete knowledge of an outbreak in order to adequately meet the reporting requirements of the WHO. While this transfer of information from provincial to federal levels could occur voluntarily, the SARS outbreak demonstrated the dangers of relying exclusively upon voluntary communication. The following comments by a federal official quoted in the Campbell report illustrate this:

> The challenge for us, nationally, was to have as much information as possible and as much information as possible that had been analyzed by Ontario, at least initially, in order to ensure that we had as complete a picture as possible of the situation in Canada, primarily in Ontario [and] that we could then share that information with other countries and with the WHO, in order to be able to demonstrate that we were responding appropriately.... I don't think we really ever felt that we were working in true partnership with the Province [Ontario].... And that inevitably led to a sense of confusion in the outside world, WHO and other countries, as to how far we had this under control.[24]

Perhaps the culmination of the evolving international health governance system is the approval of revisions to the International Health Regulations (IHR) in May 2005.[25] The new IHR, which will come into force in 2007, formally outline several responsibilities that states must assume to prepare for and respond to a public health emergency. The regulations explicitly outline that all states are required to report to the WHO, within 24 hours, any events that may be considered a public health emergency of international concern. A decision instrument in the text of the IHR provides guidance to nations to determine which public health emergencies would meet this criterion. In contrast, the previous iteration of the IHR only required reporting of three specific diseases. The new IHR also require the development of adequate surveillance capacity by all states. Within two years of the regulations coming into force, states are required to conduct an assessment of their surveillance capacity and within five years develop a public health apparatus that is fully compliant with the new IHR.

The new regulations also formalize and extend many of the powers that the WHO was utilizing during SARS. These include the authority to gather information on a possible public health emergency from all sources, as opposed to relying only upon state notifications. The WHO can share this information with other states if the affected state does not collaborate and the magnitude of the public health risk would warrant this action. The revised IHR also permit the WHO to issue both temporary and standing recommendations if an outbreak is classified as a public health emergency of international concern. These recommendations could include refusal of entry of persons from affected areas and could be made without the consent of the affected country.

The revised IHR and the new international approach to public health emergencies have important implications for Canada. To illustrate some of the governance challenges they pose, consider the possibility of a new infectious agent emerging in a Canadian province. Initial outbreak management would again be local, with supervision by the province. The revised IHR require adequate surveillance of the outbreak and communication of the status of the outbreak to the WHO officials.[26] There is a possibility, however, that the federal government may not be able to meet its reporting requirements because of a lack of intergovernmental cooperation within Canada. While the WHO would have mechanisms to obtain this data from non-governmental sources, if the WHO had to resort to such measures to monitor the outbreak, its confidence in Canada's ability to manage the outbreak would most certainly be undermined.

In this eventuality, the WHO would have the authority to issue recommendations to prevent the international spread of the disease, which could include recommending restricting travel to affected parts of Canada. Of much greater concern, of course, would be a scenario where lack of intergovernmental cooperation led to sub-optimal management of an outbreak that, in turn, contributed to the international spread of the outbreak. The danger posed by such a failure is particularly acute if, as a consequence, the outbreak spreads to a developing country. Given the lack of resources in developing countries for managing outbreaks, the spread of disease to one of these countries could be devastating for its population. If such an event occurred, Canada's intergovernmental failure would be viewed as intolerable and unacceptable from the perspective of the international health community.

INTERGOVERNMENTAL APPROACHES AND OPTIONS

As we have outlined, there are compelling reasons for stronger federal authority to manage disease outbreaks. At a minimum, detailed knowledge of the outbreak is necessary at the federal level for several reasons, including the need to (i) prepare for federal intervention in the event that the outbreak exceeds the management capacity of the province acting on its own; (ii) communicate with adjacent provinces to allow them to adequately prepare for any spread to their regions; and (iii) communicate with the international community. Additional federal powers for direct action within the confines of a province may also be required to address an outbreak that is not being managed adequately and that poses a threat to the country as a whole. Moreover, previous experience with SARS has demonstrated that Canadians cannot necessarily rely upon cordial relations among the various orders of government in times of crisis. The structure of relations between federal and provincial orders of government is thus central to Canada's capacity to manage future infectious outbreaks. In general, four broad options are available to federal officials in considering how to address this issue: a disentangled approach, a collaborative approach, an hierarchical approach, and a confederal approach.[27]

Disentangled Approach

In a "disentangled" approach to emergency public health response, federal and provincial officials would work within their own constitutionally defined areas with limited interaction. There are problems with this. First, such an approach implies there are cleanly divided constitutional responsibilities. As has been clear from analyses of public health law in Canada, however, there is considerable overlap of jurisdictional responsibilities.[28] While management of an outbreak is within the jurisdiction of a province, the potential for the outbreak to involve other provinces and the country as a whole creates a constitutional basis for federal involvement.

Second, a fundamental problem that has been consistently identified in analyses of public health in Canada has been the lack of coordination of activities among all orders of government and public health partners. Previous descriptions of public health in Canada have used the term "islands of activity" in describing the lack of coordination.[29] In doing so, these descriptions draw attention to the potential for overlap and, of more concern, gaps in critical public health functions. The disentangled approach, together with the lack of clarity on government roles and responsibilities, would perpetuate this situation and thus jeopardize the effectiveness of public health activities.

Collaborative Approach

The post-SARS approach to public health is arguably collaborative and there are clear reasons why governments at all levels — local, regional, provincial, and federal — have chosen this path. Public health requires sharing of information and coordination of activities for many of the reasons described above. Furthermore, there are real limitations on the federal government's ability to act in the absence of provincial and local cooperation, even in those areas in which the federal government has legislative authority.[30] This need for cooperation is magnified in areas such as health surveillance, where the ability of the federal government to collect data on acute and chronic diseases is clearly beyond the resources available to it on the ground.

It thus makes sense to rely, at least in part, on a collaborative approach among governments in dealing with public health emergencies. The federal government cannot afford to alienate provincial and local public health officials with a heavy-handed, top-down approach when the greatest understanding of the nature of the threat is often at the local level. However, there are also risks in assuming intergovernmental relationships will work effectively in times of crisis. In the United States, one scholar has commented that at times of crisis the different orders of government are indeed able to come together to address the challenge.[31] This was particularly evident after 9/11 (11 September 2001) and the anthrax attacks. Nevertheless, despite the extensive efforts to prepare for an emergency post-9/11, Hurricane Katrina and the flood in New Orleans revealed the susceptibility of the United States to intergovernmental jurisdictional confusion during a crisis.[32] Lack of coordination of the intergovernmental response has been blamed for contributing to preventable morbidity and mortality. Local and state officials have criticized the federal response for not providing assistance rapidly enough. Conversely, federal officials have stated that there was a lack of cooperation among state and local officials, and that the federal government had not been officially invited in — as is required under American law — at the earliest stages.[33] In light of the inadequate handling of the Hurricane Katrina emergency, the US is considering the option of federalizing emergency response, although this has provoked opposition from state officials.[34]

New Orleans should serve as a further warning to Canadian officials of the potential danger of relying *solely* upon collaborative relationships during a crisis. Regardless of which order of government had the primary responsibility to respond to the crisis and regardless of which order of government was primarily responsible for the lack of a coordinated response, to date at least, the federal government has received the majority of the blame. There appears to be an expectation that in disasters of this proportion, the responsibility to manage the crisis will be primarily federal, regardless of the constitutional division of powers and existing legislation in the area. For Canada, the lesson is straightforward. The federal government must have a contingency plan in the event of shortcomings in intergovernmental relationships. It must be able to act with great speed, since infectious diseases can spread rapidly. As already stated, we believe effective intergovernmental collaboration is the best strategy for managing an infectious outbreak, and it would be optimal if these relationships were formalized through pre-existing memoranda of understanding. We also believe, however, that Ottawa should not put all its eggs in one basket. This brings us to a third governance option.

Hierarchical Approach

As part of a contingency plan the federal government could proceed with a more hierarchical approach through a set of policy initiatives.[35] First, Ottawa could proceed with a legislative option. The federal government could amend the current emergency legislation, specifically stating that, for a public health emergency in which the properties of the crisis suggest rapid transmissibility, the federal government would have the authority to intervene without provincial permission. Alternatively, Parliament could be asked to enact new and separate emergency public health legislation that would provide the requisite authority. The merits of these different approaches are discussed later in the chapter.

Obviously, there are important limitations to the use of a federal legislative option that would need to be considered. Whatever powers the legislation provided the federal government, Ottawa would need to have the capacity to implement them. There is a question of whether the federal government has sufficient capacity, particularly with respect to the number of trained personnel, to assume command and control responsibilities in the event of an outbreak. There are also limitations on the federal capacity to enforce any power it may have on matters such as surveillance, and some level of collaboration is necessary even when the federal government has legislative authority. Therefore, questions that would need to be addressed concerning an hierarchical emergency response include the following: What existing public health personnel would Ottawa have available to assist in managing the crisis? Would the federal government have the authority to transfer public health personnel from other regions of the country to the affected region? Under what conditions could the federal government employ the Canadian Forces to carry out functions such as enforcing quarantine and distributing therapies and prophylactic measures? How exactly would the federal government structure its relations with a provincial government to maximize cooperation, given that the majority of the personnel commandeered by the federal government would be provincial?[36] The complexity of many of these issues requires that the federal government use any powers provided by legislation in a respectful manner, so as to secure the provincial and local cooperation needed for an effective response. Respectful exercise of federal powers would, for instance, dictate that the use of federal powers be restricted to appropriate circumstances and that federal actions add value to existing provincial and local efforts as opposed to simply replacing them. Just as important, the execution of such powers by the federal government should not create an excessive administrative or financial burden on the other orders of government involved.[37]

There are also other options that the federal government could consider if it chose to proceed with an hierarchical approach. One is conditional funding along the lines that the federal government has used in relation to health-care insurance under the Canada Health Transfer. In adopting this approach, the federal government could provide large block grants to provinces in exchange for their agreeing to implement certain provisions related to emergencies. These would include, most importantly, creation of surveillance infrastructure and reporting requirements for outbreaks. A provincial concern with this strategy could be that the health-care funding scenario of the 1980s and 1990s would repeat itself, with the federal government providing an increasingly smaller proportion of emergency-response funding over time.[38]

The federal government could also choose to bypass the provincial governments and interact directly with regional public health units through contracts. By doing so, it could provide seed funding to local public health units in exchange for the development of necessary programs for emergency public health response. In some ways the current model for the Public Health Agency of Canada allows for this option, although seed funding must be within the framework of an agreement with the province or territory concerned. A primary objection to this approach would be a perception that the federal government was invading provincial jurisdiction.

Confederal Approach

An intriguing alternative to federal involvement in public health emergency response is a confederal approach. This would entail provinces working together in the absence of the federal government or with the federal government as a partner, but with provincial governments having primacy.[39] Such an approach may be reasonable on a regional basis for some public health issues in which spillovers are in adjacent regions (e.g., water, air) as opposed to those issues in which spillovers are national (e.g., disease and food safety). The establishment of the Pan-Canadian Public Health Network could provide an example of the development of a confederal relationship among public health authorities across Canada.

DEFINING A NEW FEDERAL ROLE IN PUBLIC HEALTH

How, then, should the federal government proceed in defining its relations with the provinces regarding the management of public health emergencies? Inevitably relationships must be collaborative, given the importance of coordination, the recognition that local public health officials are the first line of defence against the emergency, and the general recognition of the need to share capacity. Therefore, any redefinition of a federal role must build upon and nurture the existing collaborative efforts. Furthermore, the collaborative option should be the first option considered when a public health emergency presents itself. Similarly, the federal government and provinces/territories should continue to develop national public health networks, analogous to confederal relationships, which will provide on-the-ground capacity and build the effective relationships that can be called upon at a time of crisis.

Nevertheless, even these two approaches together are not necessarily enough, and we believe that a federal "hierarchical" element needs to be incorporated into the current emergency-response strategy. While considerable effort has been undertaken to develop strong collaborative relationships, the experience with the SARS outbreak showed that the federal government cannot necessarily rely exclusively upon provincial goodwill in times of crisis. The current system needs to be insulated against the prospect of the missteps that occurred during the SARS outbreak being repeated. An additional advantage of a federal hierarchical approach is that it could further encourage provincial collaboration from the outset, which would clearly be preferable. Several issues need to be clearly outlined, however, if the federal government chooses to pursue a legislative option.

Should the Federal Government Amend the Existing Emergencies Act or Create a New Public Health Emergency Statute?

Assuming that a legislative strategy is to be pursued, two options are available to the federal government. One would simply be to amend the existing emergency legislation to make special provisions for public health emergencies that have the potential to cross provincial borders or that have already crossed international borders. The second option would be to remove public health emergencies from the existing *Emergencies Act* and deal with them in separate new public health emergency legislation. This would allow the legislation to include provisions to address the nuances of specific public health emergencies. While we have focused on the possibility of an infectious disease outbreak, other public health emergencies also present unique management challenges. Thus, separate public health emergency legislation would be able to be directed at the specific properties of the health emergency in question.

The downside of continuing to include public health emergencies in the same statute as other types of emergencies is that the public health emergency may be "tainted" by association with its potentially more draconian cousins, which are more likely to involve infringement of people's rights. And this tainting may result in the threshold for proclaiming a public health emergency being inappropriately high. Another advantage of a separate statute is that it would allow greater flexibility for tailoring federal powers and responsibilities to the nature and extent of the public health emergency as has been described in the CMA health alert system. Separate legislation would also allow distinctions to be made among the various types of public health emergencies beyond infectious diseases. All of this could be incorporated within existing legislation, but the extensive amendments required would be cumbersome within the framework of the existing statute.

Nature and Scope of Additional Powers

For the kind of public health emergency that might occur in the future, the powers embodied in the existing *Emergencies Act,* while extensive, are not sufficient. They need to be buttressed in two ways. First, as we have described, the federal government is explicitly constrained from declaring a public health emergency where the direct effects of the emergency are confined to one province unless the provincial government indicates to Ottawa that the scope of the emergency exceeds the province's capacity to deal with it. This limitation on the federal government must be removed for the simple reason that contagious diseases do not respect borders, whether internal or external. Thus, at the outset of an outbreak that could spread rapidly, the federal government should be empowered to mobilize the country's resources to aggressively intervene to break the spread of the disease. We also suggest that the federal government should be empowered to take action even if a disease is not present in any province, but is present in another country and poses a real and imminent threat of spreading to Canada. In such an instance Canadian public health officials should have the authority to take the necessary measures to prepare for the eventuality of the spread of disease to Canada, including the mobilization of appropriate personnel, the distribution of preventative and therapeutic medicines and the institution of appropriate surveillance measures.

Second, the federal government must possess the authority to demand timely information from other orders of government. The current *Emergencies Act* does not explicitly grant that authority to Ottawa. If the federal authorities can track the pattern of disease migration, they will know whether additional powers must be proclaimed and in which areas of the country they will be needed. This kind of information flow between the Ontario and federal authorities was lacking during the SARS crisis in 2003. This additional power may raise privacy issues that will have to be worked through in a manner that recognizes competing claims for the public good.

Conditions under which the Federal Government would be Authorized to Invoke Emergency Public Health Powers

The new or amended federal legislation should be precise about the conditions under which federal emergency powers can be invoked. We suggest that the decision to permit federal involvement be guided by the fundamental properties of the infectious threat. Federal action would be justified if the following criteria were met: (i) there is clear potential for cross-border transmission; (ii) the health consequences of the epidemic are potentially severe; and (iii) a national approach to controlling the outbreak could be reasonably considered to be more effective than a purely local approach.

Further guidance could be drawn from the WHO's decision instrument for the assessment and notification of events constituting a public health emergency of international concern (Figure 1). Member nations are expected to apply this instrument to developing outbreaks within their borders. Events that constitute a public health emergency of international concern must meet at least two of the following criteria: (i) the public health impact of the event is serious; (ii) the event is unusual or unexpected; (iii) there is a significant risk of international spread; and (iv) there is a significant risk of international travel or trade restrictions. Modifying this instrument for events of national concern and incorporating it within Canadian legislation would have two advantages. First, it would reassure provincial governments that the federal government would not use any new powers arbitrarily. Second, it would assist Canada in meeting the requirements of the revised International Health Regulations, thereby meeting our international commitments as well as potentially protecting us from the WHO travel recommendations.

FIGURE 1

Decision Instrument for the Assessment and Notification of Events that May Constitute a Public Health Emergency of International Concern

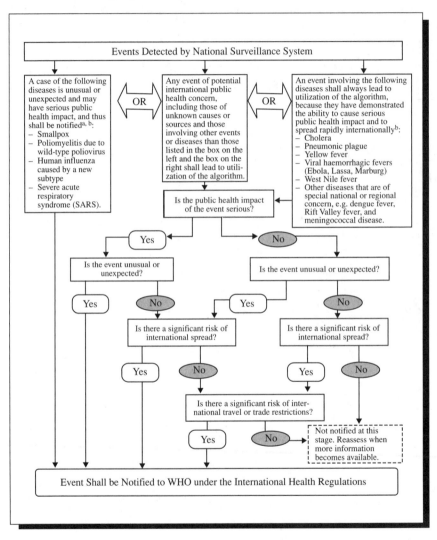

Notes: [a] As per the WHO case definitions.

[b] The disease list shall be used only for the purposes of these Regulations.

Source: World Health Organization (WHO), Third Report of Committee A. Fifty-eighth World Health Assembly, Agenda Item 13.1 (Geneva: WHO, 2005), Annex 2.

Funding the Costs of a Public Health Emergency

Given that a public health emergency is of national interest, the incremental cost of dealing with an emergency should be disproportionately borne by the federal authorities. And, the larger and more costly the emergency, the greater the share that the federal government should bear. Fundamentally, it would appear appropriate to distribute the cost of responding to a public health crisis such as an epidemic, which would have the potential to cross provincial lines, across all Canadian taxpayers. Residents in Manitoba, for example, would have a clear interest in having their tax dollars devoted to controlling an outbreak in a region of Ontario that approaches their border.

In the context of the institution of a graded emergency-response system within separate public health emergency legislation, we support the CMA's vision that the greater the level of the emergency the greater the federal government responsibility for funding the emergency response. For example, at the earliest level of an emergency, the federal government might simply require transfer of information in a timely manner and would provide funding to assist with collection of data. In the presence of a full-blown outbreak that is potentially of a national scale, the federal government might assume command-and-control authority and would therefore be responsible for providing some measure of compensation to public health officials and health-care workers whose services they employ. The introduction of a graded funding system to parallel the graded emergency-alert system would have the benefit of preventing the federal government from abusing its new powers since it would have to consider the potential financial cost of any decision to use them. In contrast, the failure to implement such a system could create unfunded mandates at the provincial level that could have serious economic consequences for the province, which may not have the resources to respond to federal demands, as well as damage future intergovernmental relationships.

Constraining the Federal Emergency Authority

Part VI of the *Emergencies Act* sets out the rules for parliamentary supervision of an emergency declaration. It requires the federal government to table a motion in Parliament within seven sitting days after the emergency has been proclaimed. Each house is required to debate the motion on the sitting day after the sitting day on which the motion was laid before the House and to debate it uninterrupted until it is ready for a vote. A negative vote by either House puts an end to the emergency declaration. Part VI of the act also requires Parliament to consider a motion from either 20 MPs or ten senators to debate a proposed revocation of all or part of the emergency declaration. There are also provisions for all orders and regulations to be laid before Parliament within two sitting days after they are made. Parliament's existing supervisory powers seem to us to be sufficient to deal with the proposed enlarged powers that would be assigned to the federal government.

FEASIBILITY OF OUR APPROACH

The primary concern about the legislative and governance strategy we have proposed is that it could be viewed as being inconsistent with the current approach to public health that is centred on collaboration. Of more practical concern is the argument that in the absence of provincial cooperation the ability of the federal government to act is limited, even with the requisite legislative authority. Thus, any new federal powers would be functionally meaningless. These are potentially important limitations and worth considering in more detail.

Public health officials, when developing a plan for a new public health agency, did consider the option of a federal command-and-control approach to public health emergencies. However, this was dismissed for several reasons, primarily centring on several issues we have previously discussed: the importance of local response and the danger of conflict between local and regional officials, who have the knowledge and resources to act, and federal officials, who may have the legislative authority to act. In particular, given a scenario where a province refuses to allow federal intervention, what then would be the federal option? It would be both challenging and disruptive for the federal government to commandeer local health workers for federal purposes under these circumstances. Such an action would almost certainly create problems in the "on-the-ground" response to the emergency.

While these concerns are very real, they do not invalidate our argument. Our starting premise has always been to recognize the necessity of a collaborative approach. We have argued that in the presence of a federal legislative backup option, the willingness of provinces to collaborate from the outset is greater. Furthermore, the problems of provincial lack of cooperation would still apply under existing legislation, the primary difference being that the potential for conflict would only occur when the emergency involved two provinces. Our argument is that the test for federal authority should not be governed by political borders, but rather the nature of the national or international threat posed by a pathogen. In our view, it is scientifically inconsistent to argue that the federal government should have clearly defined authority to control an outbreak that involves two provinces but that it should have no role at the outset of an outbreak, when the potential benefit of a federal response is the greatest. Further demonstrating the problems with the current state of affairs is the fact that a public health emergency could be declared by the WHO to be of international concern but not merit federal jurisdiction under our current governance strategy.

A second rationale for our proposal for an alternative test for federal action is that we believe it would be more difficult for a province to refuse federal involvement in the presence of federal legislative authority. There is a distinction to be drawn between the passive action of a province not inviting the federal government in, as would be the case at present, to actively refusing federal participation. In the second scenario, a province is accepting a large political risk if its public views the provincial efforts to have been inadequate and are aware that the provincial authorities actively rejected federal involvement.

An intriguing question remains as to what the federal government would do if a public health emergency did arise within a province and relations between the federal government and the province broke down. One option available to Ottawa might be to send in the Canadian Forces to seize control of public health personnel and capacity. This scenario likely would be more harmful than beneficial and almost certainly should not occur. An alternative would be to take measures to protect the rest of the country from spread of disease from the non-compliant province. This would include recommending travel bans to and from the affected province, including preventing flights into and out of the province. While this option would be politically dangerous and practically challenging, in the event of a full-fledged pandemic, it would have to be strongly considered. If the federal government fails to do so, the WHO would in essence make the decision for Ottawa, by issuing a travel advisory to the affected region.

What we have argued is not meant to be a statement that the federal government is, at present, more qualified to handle public health emergencies than other orders of government. Our recommendations would place a burden of responsibility on the federal government to have the capacity to adequately respond. At this time, that may be a burden it may wish not to have because of the investment it would require as well as the political risk with which it would be associated. On the other hand, we have previously stated that a lesson from Katrina may be that the public assumes it is the federal government's responsibility to address emergencies of that magnitude, even if they are not in the federal jurisdiction. A second lesson from Katrina is that when the federal government is asked to act, its response must be adequate. If not, the public's confidence in the federal government to protect them from future threats will be greatly weakened.

POTENTIAL HUMAN AVIAN FLU PANDEMIC

The obvious application of the governance strategy we have proposed is to the management of a potential human avian flu pandemic. At present, international efforts are being taken to prepare for an expected human influenza pandemic from the H5N1 virus. This virus has been demonstrated to have both a high level of pathogenicity as well as potential for mutation. Infections with the H5N1 virus have primarily been restricted to birds and the development of highly pathogenic strains of the virus in birds have created epidemics with mortality rates of close to 100 percent.[40] Occasional bird-to-human transmission has occurred and is a point of growing concern. As of 6 March 2006, 175 human cases of H5N1 infection had been identified and 95 of these cases resulted in death, a mortality rate of just over 50 percent.[41] These human cases have been restricted to Cambodia, China, Indonesia, Thailand, Vietnam, Iraq, and Turkey. As avian H5N1 infections spread throughout the world, an increasing number of bird-to-human transmissions are expected to occur and will likely extend beyond these countries.

The key variable that is currently not present for a pandemic is the ability for the pathogen to travel from human to human. If the virus were to mutate into a human-to-human transmissible form, public health officials fear a catastrophic spread of the disease worldwide. The WHO and most nations have developed pandemic plans to prepare for such an event. The key components of these plans include: aggressive disease surveillance, early identification of human-to-human transmission, timely communication with the WHO, and the aggressive institution of measures to prevent a spread including development and distribution of an effective vaccine, distribution of the antiviral oseltamavir (Tamiflu) and the appropriate use of social distancing measures.

A potential influenza pandemic has been of considerable concern for Canadian public health officials. The official federal plan estimates that, in the event of a pandemic, 4.5 to 10.6 million Canadians would become clinically ill, 34,000 to 180,000 will require hospitalization and 11,000 to 58,000 deaths could be expected. The plan outlines which order of government is to be responsible for specific functions (e.g., surveillance, information-sharing, vaccines, antivirals, health services) during each phase of the pandemic. The roles and responsibilities are primarily shared, recognizing the need for a collaborative approach to managing the emergency. While the plan states that the federal government is the lead in some of the collaborative responses it does not describe the exact authority and powers that would be available to the federal government.[42]

The planned response to a human avian flu outbreak in Canada has many characteristics that could result in intergovernmental conflict and a sub-optimal response. There would be pressures for a province to not report at the outset because of concerns about the impact on its poultry industry and on tourism. As described, earlier simulations have also suggested that a rapid response involving all of the country's resources would be required to stop the spread of disease and that this is not necessarily guaranteed. We would expect in the event of a Canadian human avian flu outbreak that orders of government would work together in a collaborative manner, primarily because of the attention focused on the issue and the intense scrutiny any response would receive. It is during the unexpected emergencies, SARS and Katrina for example, where the possibility for many of the intergovernmental problems we have described to arise is greatest. However, even in the presence of well thought-out plans, such as with avian flu, we believe that response could benefit from a backup approach that takes into consideration the possibility of intergovernmental sluggishness or even a dispute arising during the response. Given the magnitude of the morbidity and mortality expected with the outbreak, every measure should be taken to ensure that Canadians can protect themselves against the kinds of disputes that arose during the SARS crisis. In the case of avian flu the consequences of such disputes are likely to be considerably greater.

CONCLUSION

Ensuring that this country is prepared for the next pandemic is a high priority for public health officials. We would again like to emphasize that establishing the necessary public health infrastructure and capacity is of central importance in preparing for this threat. However, a critical component of any such preparation will also be to guarantee that effective relationships exist among the various orders of government that will need to work together to manage the emergency. We have argued that an essential component of developing effective relationships is to establish a strong federal role in the emergency-response process. Strong federal leadership is essential to ensure that communication exists among provinces and with the international community. This will allow adjacent provinces and other countries to take the appropriate measures to prepare for the possible transmission of disease to their populations. It will also allow Canada to meet the requirements of the new International Health Regulations and protect itself from the avoidable introduction of travel advisories or restrictions that could have a devastating effect on regional economies.

We believe that the issues described in this chapter, which have also been identified in previous reports, should be addressed urgently. Doing so will both enhance Canada's ability to respond to a potential flu pandemic and allow us to fulfill our international responsibilities.

NOTES

This research was funded by grants from the Canadian Institutes of Health Research. Dr. Wilson is supported as a New Investigator by the Canadian Institutes of Health Research.

[1]Kumanan Wilson, "A Canadian Agency for Public Health: Could it Work?" *Canadian Medical Association Journal* 170, no. 2 (2004):222-23.

[2]Vivek Goel, "What Do We Do with the SARS Reports?" *Healthcare Quarterly* 7 (2004):28-41.

[3]World Health Organization (WHO), "WHO Extends its SARS-related Travel Advice to Beijing and Shanxi Province in China and to Toronto Canada," Update No. 37 (Geneva: WHO, 2003); T. Svoboda, B. Henry, L. Shulman, E. Kennedy, E. Rea, W. Ng, T. Wallington, B. Yaffe, E. Gournis, E. Vicencio, S. Basrur and R.H. Glazier, "Public Health Measures to Control the Spread of the Severe Acute Respiratory Syndrome during the Outbreak in Toronto," *New England Journal of Medicine* 350, no. 23 (2004):2352-61.

[4]R.P. Wenzel and M.B. Edmond, "Managing SARS amidst Uncertainty," *New England Journal of Medicine* 348, no. 20 (2003):1947-48.

[5]Brad Mackay, "Toronto Quarantines Patients as SARS Concern Grows," *e-CMAJ* 26 March 2003. Ontario declared that SARS was a communicable and virulent disease. This allowed the chief medical officer of health, under the *Health Protection and Promotion Act*, to "by a written order ... require a person to take or to refrain from taking any action that is specified in the order in respect of a communicable disease" (*Health Protection and Promotion Act*, R.S.O. 1990, c. H.7, s. 22(1)). Such orders include "requiring any person that the order states has or may have a communicable disease or is or may be infected with an agent of a communicable disease to isolate himself or herself and remain in isolation from other persons" (*Health Protection Act*, s. 22(4) (c)).

[6]The National Advisory Committee on SARS and Public Health, "SARS in Canada: Anatomy of an Outbreak," in *Learning from SARS: Renewal of Public Health in Canada* (Ottawa: Health Canada, 2003), ch. 2.

[7]R.S. 1985 (4th Supp.), c. 22 (hereinafter cited as the *Emergencies Act*).

[8]R.S. 1985 (4th Supp.), c. 6 (hereinafter cited as the *Emergency Preparedness Act*).

[9]*Emergencies Act*, s. 14(2).

[10]British Columbia reported four probable cases of SARS. Only one of these was proven to be a case of secondary transmission within the province, the others occurring in returning travelers. The lack of community spread of SARS in British Columbia differentiated it substantially from Toronto, and the outbreak would not have been considered an "emergency."

[11]Independent SARS Commission (Mr. Justice Archie Campbell, chair), "Problem 7: Poor Coordination with Federal Government," in *SARS and Public Health in Ontario*, Interim Report (Toronto: Government of Ontario, 2004).

[12]C. Alphonso and G. York, "Canadian Health Officials Rapped by WHO," *The Globe and Mail* (National Edition), 13 June 2003, pp. A1, A6.

[13]The National Advisory Committee on SARS and Public Health, "Executive Summary," in *Learning from SARS*; The Standing Senate Committee on Social Affairs, Science and Technology (Michael Kirby, Chair), *Reforming Health Protection and Promotion in Canada: Time to Act* (Ottawa: Standing Senate Committee on Social Affairs, Science and Technology, 2003).

[14]Canadian Medical Association, "CMA Submission on Infrastructure and Governance of the Public Health System in Canada." Presentations to the Senate Standing Committee on Social Affairs, Science and Technology, 2003.

[15]The National Advisory Committee on SARS and Public Health, "Some Legal and Ethical Issues Raised by SARS and Infectious Diseases in Canada," in *Learning from SARS*, ch. 9.

[16]Privy Council Office, *Securing an Open Society: Canada's National Security Policy* (Ottawa: Privy Council Office, 2004).

[17]N.M. Ferguson, D.A. Cummings, S. Cauchemez, C. Fraser, S. Riley, A. Meeyai, S. Iamsirithaworn and D.S. Burke, "Strategies for Containing an Emerging Influenza Pandemic in Southeast Asia," *Nature* 437, no. 7056 (2005):209-14; I.M. Longini, Jr., A. Nizam, S. Xu, K. Ungchusak, W. Hanshaoworakul, D.A. Cummings and M.E. Halloran. "Containing Pandemic Influenza at the Source," *Science* 309, no. 5737 (2005):1083-87.

[18]David P. Fidler, "Germs, Governance, and Global Public Health in the Wake of SARS," *Journal of Clinical Investigation* 113, no. 6 (2004):799-804; David P. Fidler, "Emerging Trends in International Law Concerning Global Infectious Disease Control," *Emerging Infectious Diseases* 9, no. 3 (2003):285-90; Lawrence Gostin, "The International Health Regulations and Beyond," *Lancet Infectious Diseases* 4, no. 10 (2004):606-07; Ilona Kickbusch, "The Development of International Health Policies: Accountability Intact?" *Social Science & Medicine* 51, no. 6 (2000):979-89.

[19]David P. Fidler, "SARS: Political Pathology of the First Post-Westphalian Pathogen," *Journal of Law, Medicine & Ethics* 31, no. 4 (2003):485-505.

[20]World Health Organization, *Global Crises, Global Solutions: Managing Public Health Emergencies of International Concern through the Revised International Health Regulations* (Geneva: WHO, 2002).

[21]Public Health Agency of Canada, *What is the Global Public Health Intelligence Network (GPHIN)?* 2004 [cited 4 October 2005]. At www.phac-aspc.gc.ca/media/nr-rp/2004/2004_gphin-rmispbk_e.html. Of note, GPHIN provided the earliest evidence of a respiratory outbreak in Guangdong Province in China.

[22]Fidler, "Germs, Governance, and Global Public Health in the Wake of SARS."

[23]World Health Organization, "WHO Extends its SARS-related Travel Advice to Beijing and Shanxi Province in China and to Toronto Canada."

[24]Independent SARS Commission, *SARS and Public Health in Ontario* (Toronto: Government of Ontario, 2004), pp. 66, 68.

[25]World Health Organization, "WHO Extends its SARS-related Travel Advice to Beijing and Shanxi Province in China and to Toronto Canada."

[26]Ibid.

[27]Harvey Lazar and Tom MacIntosh, *Federalism, Democracy and Social Policy: Towards a Sectoral Approach to the Social Union* (Kingston: Institute of Intergovernmental Relations, Queen's University, 1998).

[28]M. Jackman, "The Constitutional Basis for Federal Regulation of Health," *Health Law Review* 5, no. 2 (1996):3-10; A. Braen, "Health and the Distribution of Powers in Canada," in *Commission on the Future of Health Care in Canada* (Ottawa: National Library of Canada, 2002).

[29]Kumanan Wilson, "The Role of Federalism in Health Surveillance: A Case Study of the National Health-Surveillance 'Infostructure,'" in *Federalism, Democracy and Health Policy in Canada*, ed. Duane Adams (Kingston: Institute of Intergovernmental Relations, Queen's University, 2001).

[30]The federal government's call to stop sales of the natural health product Kava was not observed by several health food stores in the Toronto area. The ability to

police all health food stores would be beyond the federal government's capacity, and provincial assistance would be required in the policing efforts.

[31]W.E. Parmet, "After September 11: Rethinking Public Health Federalism," *Journal of Law, Medicine & Ethics* 30, no. 2 (2002):201-11.

[32]"Katrina Reveals Fatal Weaknesses in US Public Health," Editorial, *Lancet* 366, no. 9489 (2005):867.

[33]D. Stout, "Former FEMA Chief Blames Local Officials for Failures," *New York Times*, 27 September 2005.

[34]J. Bush, "Think Locally on Relief," *Washington Post*, 30 September 2005, p. A19.

[35]In this paper we use the term *hierarchical* to describe a set of intergovernmental relations where one order of government is able to enforce its mandate on another order of government. We recognize the somewhat normative nature of this term and would like to emphasize that hierarchical relationships and cordial relationships are not mutually exclusive.

[36]The federal SARS report comments that the Federal/Provincial/Territorial Network for Emergency Preparedness and Response has worked toward establishing health emergency response teams (HERTs) that could provide additional support in the event of an outbreak. President Bush has recently announced that in the event of an avian flu outbreak in the US, he would consider utilizing the military to enforce quarantine.

[37]Ontario's then minister of health, Minister Clement, was quoted in the SARS Commission's interim report as saying, "We felt we were giving all of the information that we had available to us in an immediate way. But we were unaware of exactly how that was being transmitted to the WHO, or the requirements of the WHO for the type of information required.... They [Health Canada] didn't take it seriously at our borders, they didn't take it seriously in terms of the requirements that we needed in terms of resources. That's a matter of public record."

[38]Kumanan Wilson, "Health Care, Federalism and the New Social Union," *Canadian Medical Association Journal* 162, no. 8 (2000):1171-74.

[39]Thomas J. Courchene, "ACCESS: A Convention on the Canadian Economic and Social Systems." Paper presented at "Assessing ACCESS: Towards a New Social Union" symposium on the Courchene proposal, Kingston, 1997.

[40]World Health Organization. "WHO Extends its SARS-related Travel Advice to Beijing and Shanxi Province in China and to Toronto Canada."

[41]World Health Organization. *Cumulative Number of Confirmed Human Cases of Avian Influenza A/(H5N1) Reported to WHO*. 6 March 2006 [cited 9 March 2006]. At www.who.int/csr/disease/avian_influenza/country/cases_table_2006_03_06/en/index.html.

[42]Public Health Agency of Canada, *Canadian Pandemic Influenza Plan* (Ottawa: Health Canada, 2004). At www.phac-aspc.gc.ca/cpip-pclcpi/.

11

THE ECONOMIC IMPACTS OF SARS AND PANDEMIC INFLUENZA

Steven James and Timothy Sargent

INTRODUCTION

The SARS outbreak in 2003 and the current threat from the H5N1 avian flu virus have led to a great deal of concern in public health circles. There are fears that the H5N1 virus will mutate into a form that could be transmissible among humans, and that this new virus could spark an influenza pandemic possibly as severe as that observed in 1918. Much of the focus has been on the human cost of such a crisis, which is certainly very substantial. However, it has also prompted governments, business interests, economists, and the general population to speculate about the economic impacts of pandemics. Many studies have argued that a pandemic could have large negative economic impacts. Sherry Cooper, for example, predicts that a mild pandemic would reduce global gross domestic product (GDP) by 2 percent while a severe pandemic would reduce GDP by 6 percent, and that "depending on its length and severity, its economic impact could be comparable, at least for a short time, to the Great Depression of the 1930s."[1]

This concern about the economic impacts of a potential pandemic stems in part from a perception that in the last few years fundamentally non-economic shocks such as the 9/11 (11 September 2001) terrorist attacks and the outbreak of SARS have had important economic impacts at the macroeconomic level. For example, Bloom, de Wit and Carangel-San Jose argue that "the outbreak of SARS in 2003 showed that even a disease with a relatively small health impact can have a major economic impact."[2] This makes it very important for economists to understand exactly how and to what extent infectious diseases affect the economy. In this study we attempt to do precisely that by looking at economic data from the SARS outbreak in 2003, and from the three major influenza pandemics of the twentieth century: 1918, 1957, and 1968. We will also touch briefly on the impacts of 9/11. In each case we will review the historical evidence and attempt to assess whether, in fact, there were noticeable impacts on the overall economy of the countries affected.

THE ECONOMIC IMPACT OF SARS

SARS was an atypical pneumonia that first appeared in China in late 2002. The disease reached Hong Kong and Vietnam in February 2003, and then spread to other countries in the spring. The World Health Organization (WHO) estimates that 8,096 people were infected, of whom 774 died, implying a case mortality rate of 9.6 percent.[3] This compares with more than 10 million cases and 40,000 deaths from influenza globally in an average non-pandemic year. Canada was the most affected non-Asian country with 251 cases and 44 deaths, most of these in Toronto. About 3,500 people were quarantined in Hong Kong, Singapore, and Taiwan, and many more in Canada. Schools were closed in Hong Kong and Singapore. The WHO recommended the screening of airline passengers and advised against all but essential travel to Toronto.

The Macroeconomic Impact of SARS in Asia

Hong Kong — at the epicentre of SARS — suffered a real GDP decline in the second quarter of 2003; however, this barely stands out relative to the typical volatility of Hong Kong GDP (Figure 1). This decline is fully explained by a fall in service exports (likely travel services) (Figure 2). Annual tourist visits are equal to 203 percent of Hong Kong's population compared with 4 percent for an economy like Japan, making total Hong Kong GDP much more vulnerable to reductions in visits from abroad. Service exports rebounded in the subsequent quarter while goods exports were unaffected. Air cargo shipments continued unabated even as personal air travel fell sharply.

Restaurant revenues dipped a surprisingly small 10 percent in the quarter (Figure 3), with this fall likely partly a result of reduced travel to Hong Kong. Hong Kong retail sales actually rose as SARS cases surged in March 2003 (Figure 4), at odds with Lee and McKibbin's assumption of a 15 percent

FIGURE 1

Hong Kong and Singapore: Real GDP, 2000–2005 (2000 Q1 = 100; sa)

FIGURE 2

Hong Kong: Real Export and Import Growth, 2000–2005 (y/y)

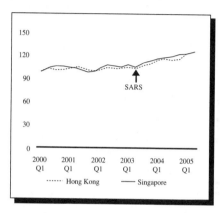

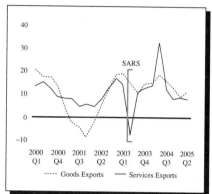

Note: Here and in subsequent figures, seasonally adjusted is denoted "sa"; year over year changes are denoted "y/y"; Quarter is denoted "Q."

Source: All figures used in this chapter are authors' compilation.

FIGURE 3

Hong Kong: Real Restaurant Receipts, 2000–2005 (Index; sa)

FIGURE 4

Hong Kong: Real Retail Sales, 2002–2004 (Index; sa)

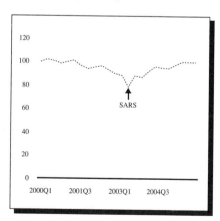

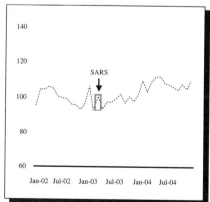

Note: See note to Figure 1.

decline lasting six months.[4] Alan Siu and Richard Wong find that the Hong Kong economy "did not experience a supply shock, as the manufacturing base in the Pearl River Delta was unaffected, and goods continued to be exported through Hong Kong normally." They add that "initial alarmist reports about the negative economic impacts were not borne out."[5]

SARS struck Singapore in March and April of 2003. Visits plunged in April and remained depressed in May, before beginning a sharp rebound in June (Figure 5). Hotel occupancy fell from 71 percent in March to 34 percent in April. The quarterly GDP pattern is similar to that of Hong Kong. As in Hong Kong, retail sales were completely unaffected, and shipping tonnage and freight carried by Singapore airlines actually rose during the height of SARS.

FIGURE 5

Singapore: Real Retail Sales, Visitor Arrivals, Shipping Tonnage, and
Airline Freight Carried, 2002–2004
(Jan 2001 = 100)

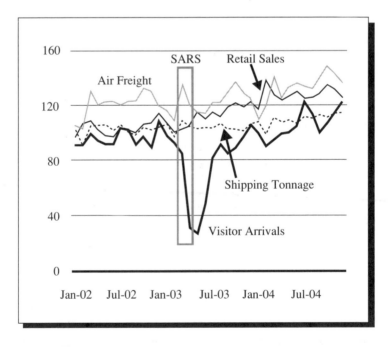

Note: See note to Figure 1.

SARS impacts are not apparent in the annual growth patterns of Hong Kong, China, and Vietnam (Table 1). All three economies experienced faster growth in 2003 than in 2002. Only in Singapore did annual growth slow in 2003.

TABLE 1

Real GDP Growth: Asian Countries Affected by SARS, 2000–2004

	Hong Kong (%)	China (%)	Singapore (%)	Vietnam (%)
2000	10.2	8.0	9.6	6.8
2001	0.5	7.5	−2.0	6.9
2002	1.9	8.3	3.2	7.1
2003	3.2	9.5	1.4	7.3
2004	8.1	9.5	8.4	7.7

The Macroeconomic Impact of SARS in Canada

Real GDP declined in Canada in the second quarter of 2003. Newcomb has cited this as evidence that SARS had a significant negative impact on the Canadian economy.[6] A deeper analysis of the data does not support this conclusion.

Real net exports of travel services declined in the SARS quarter and have remained well below pre-SARS levels since then (Figure 6). At first glance, this seems to support the idea of a significant and even long-lasting impact. However, this apparent correlation is deceptive as it ignores the role played by the unprecedented appreciation of the Canadian dollar against the US dollar in the second quarter of 2003 (Figure 7). This appreciation fully explains the decline in net exports of travel services, with the residual from a regression of net exports of travel services on the real Canada-US exchange rate showing no role for SARS.[7]

Figure 8 shows that SARS had no apparent impact on the output of either the transit and ground transport industry or the food service and drinking place industry. In Ontario — dominated by Toronto, the city most affected by SARS — retail sales and restaurant receipts actually grew faster during the outbreak than in the rest of Canada (Figure 9). While anecdotal reports at the time suggested that these sectors were significantly affected by SARS, the hard

FIGURE 6

Canadian Real Exports and Imports of
Travel Services, 2000–2005

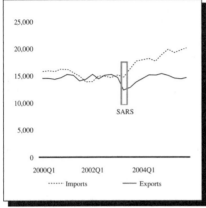

Note: See note to Figure 1.

FIGURE 7

Net Trade in Travel Services Not Explained
by the Real Exchange Rate, 1981–2005

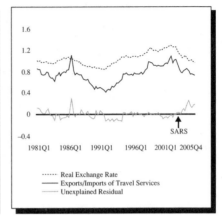

FIGURE 8

Canadian Industry GDP at Basic Prices,
2001–2005

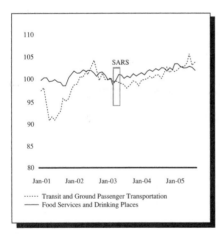

Note: See note to Figure 1.

FIGURE 9

Retail Sales and Restaurant Receipts,
Ontario/Rest of Canada, Indices,
2002–2005

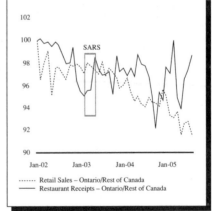

data do not support this. Some individual firms may have been affected, but not enough to show up in the aggregate data.

The output of the air transportation and accommodation industry fell 14 percent between March and May 2003, while accommodation output fell 8 percent (Figure 10), with the accommodation decline likely resulting from re-duced travel. Much of this doubtless reflected fear by international travellers of flying to Toronto during the outbreak; however, a significant portion may have been unrelated to SARS. The SARS outbreak coincided with the start of the second Gulf War and heightened fears of terrorist attacks. As Figure 11 shows, US global air travel declined sharply at the time of the first Gulf War. Similar impacts are apparent when the second Gulf War began, with travel to Atlantic and Pacific destinations affected equally. This suggests that most of the decline in US international travel in the spring of 2003 reflected a general-ized fear of terrorism, not SARS. If SARS had been the principal cause then we would have expected to see a much greater impact on travel to Pacific des-tinations than to Atlantic destinations. In the case of travel to Canada we cannot easily disentangle SARS from heightened fear of terrorism, and it is likely that both played a role in the reduction in air travel during this period.

FIGURE 10
Canadian Industry GDP at Basic Prices,
2001–2005

FIGURE 11
US Air Travel by Region, 1988–2005

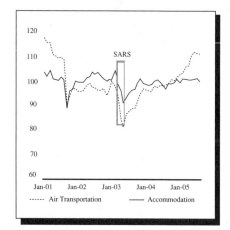

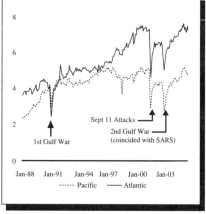

Note: See note to Figure 1.

The reduction in Canadian travel services and accommodation output between March and May equals 0.03 percent of 2003 GDP. While much of this may have stemmed from SARS, some likely reflected a generalized fear of international air travel at the time of the second Gulf War.

Fan says that the "pronounced impact of SARS" can be attributed to "the almost costless and rapid transmission of information due to the development of modern media and communications technologies."[8] McKibbin and Sidorenko develop assumptions regarding the psychological effects of an influenza pandemic using a framework that is identical to that developed by Lee and McKibbin in their analysis of SARS.[9] Lee and McKibbin express the essence of this framework as:

> First, fear of SARS infection leads to a substantial decline in consumer demand, especially for travel and retail sales service. The fast speed of contagion makes people avoid social interaction. The adverse demand shock becomes more substantial in the regions which have much larger service-related activities and higher population densities, such as Hong Kong or Beijing, China. The psychological shock ripples all around the world ... since the world is so closely linked by international travel. Second, the uncertain features of the disease reduces confidence in the future of the affected economies ... the loss of foreign investors' confidence would potentially have tremendous impacts on foreign investment flows.[10]

Our reading of the evidence leads us to quite different conclusions regarding the lessons of SARS. The hard data suggest that SARS had one economic impact — namely, a temporary reduction in international travel to affected locations, with some associated impacts on accommodation. No other impacts are apparent in either South Asia or Canada. Goods trade, supply chains, and retail sales were all unaffected.

We do not know what the state of mind was of people living in locations affected by SARS. Survey data from Taiwan suggest that they were fearful and uneasy — just as people in 1918 likely were on a much greater scale.[11] Nevertheless, their behaviour did not change in ways that led to observable economic impacts.

THE ECONOMIC IMPACTS OF THE TERRORIST ATTACKS OF 9/11

McKibbin and Sidorenko argue that "the fear of an unknown deadly virus is similar in its psychological effects to the reaction to bio- and other terrorism threats." We have no data to refute or support this, however, we would agree that the behavioural effects of an event like the 9/11 terrorist attacks resemble those of SARS. US passenger transportation dropped sharply in the wake of 9/11 (Figure 12). Not surprisingly, air passenger transportation was particularly hit, but personal vehicle transportation across the Canada-US land border also dropped noticeably. However, freight transportation was essentially unaffected. Even air freight transportation suffered a surprisingly small decline given that air traffic was actually halted for a period after the attacks.

US retail sales dropped slightly in September 2001 and automobile sales fell modestly (Figure 13). This may or may not have been because people felt uneasy or depressed following the attacks. However, as Albala-Bertrand stresses, people operating in market economies are not passive in the face of disasters.[12] Automobile dealers responded to the perceived demand weakness by offering 0 percent financing of new purchases. This led to close to a 25 percent surge in automobile sales in October that dwarfed the September decline. At the time of 9/11 many feared a blow to consumer confidence that would tip the United States back into a protracted recession. The data suggest that the market response to the attacks ensured that the actual effect on cumulative retail sales over the September to December period was positive rather than negative.

FIGURE 12

US: Transportation Services Index, 1990–2005

FIGURE 13

US: Retail Sales, 2001–2002

(nominal, sa, Aug 2001 = 100)

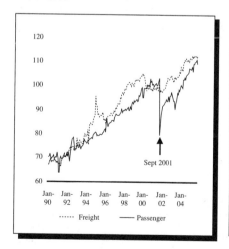

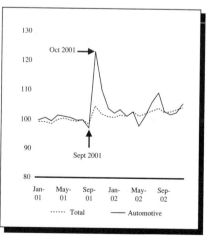

Note: See note to Figure 1.

The behavioural responses to SARS and 9/11 share a common feature. In both cases, people temporarily avoided air travel as a risk-reduction strategy. In the case of SARS, they avoided travelling to the locus of infection. After 9/11 they avoided a mode of travel that they suddenly perceived as riskier. However, what they did not do is as interesting as what they did do. Those who actually lived in Hong Kong, Singapore, Taiwan, and Toronto did not "hunker down" or flee in panic. Rather, they carried on with their lives, including working and shopping. They may have been anxious — 50 percent of Taiwan respondents reported wearing a mask during the height of SARS — but they did not become paralysed with fear, even in the face of intense media coverage.

The difference between international travellers and the residents of the affected locations is that the former could easily avoid the perceived risk, whereas the latter could not. A risk that is pervasive and hard to avoid engenders coping strategies that enable people to continue functioning. These strategies involve selective processing of information that reduces the disutility associated with anxiety regarding the risk. Their importance is stressed in an emerging literature that merges insights from psychology and economics.[13] When a risk is pervasive, the relative risk associated with particular activities will also tend to shrink.

THE ECONOMIC IMPACTS OF INFLUENZA PANDEMICS

There have been three influenza pandemics during the past one hundred years: 1918, 1957, and 1968. Morbidity rates (the proportion of the population experiencing symptoms) ranged between 20 and 35 percent, and many more were likely infected but asymptomatic. While high infection rates were common to these three pandemics, resulting mortality differed greatly. The 1918 pandemic featured much higher mortality than the 1957 and 1968 pandemics. Case mortality rates in 1957 and 1968 did not differ much from those of normal winter epidemic influenza.

There is thus no generic pandemic, either in terms of mortality or economic consequences. A pandemic could be associated with high mortality as in 1918, or low mortality as in 1957 and 1968, or something very different.

While past pandemics have featured several waves of morbidity, most cases have been concentrated in a single wave lasting no more than six to eight weeks in any given location. This would likely be the only wave with any noticeable economic effects.

The Economic Impact of the 1918 Pandemic

The 1918 influenza pandemic was far more severe than any other for which we have reliable data. About 20 to 25 percent of North Americans fell ill between September 1918 and January 1919. US case mortality ranged between 1.75 and 2.25 percent, with half the deaths occurring in the month of October (Figure 14).

FIGURE 14
US: Excess Mortality Rate, 1914–1919
(per 1,000)

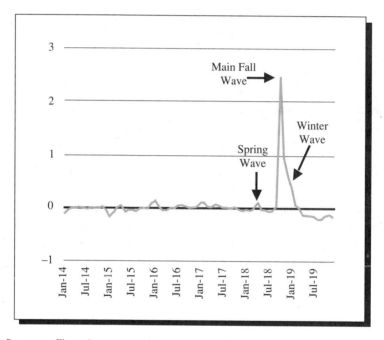

Note: See note to Figure 1.

Mortality in 1918 was unusually great in the 20-to-40 age group (Figure 15) with males disproportionately affected. The impact on the labour force would thus have been greater than in standard influenza epidemics that disproportionately affect the very young and the very old. The mortality spike at age 35 did not reflect a higher attack rate, but rather a spike in pneumonia as a secondary complication (Figure 16).

FIGURE 15

Age-Specific Influenza and Pneumonia
Excess Mortality: United States, 1918
(per 100,000 per year)

FIGURE 16

Age-Specific Influenza and Pneumonia
Attack Rate: Baltimore, Maryland,
September 1918 to January 1919
(per 1,000 per year)

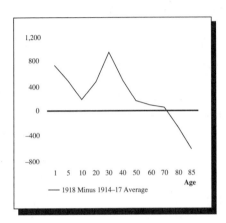

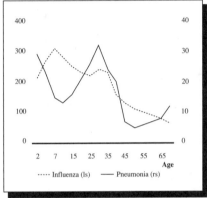

Note: See note to Figure 1. ls = left hand side; rs = right hand side.

While official US Bureau of Economic Analysis (BEA) GDP estimates do not exist prior to 1929, the National Bureau of Economic Research (NBER) Macro History Database provides a rich source of high frequency data to analyze the economic impact of the 1918 pandemic. Monthly data for the production of a wide variety of commodities are available, as well as goods trade data, data on the consumption of travel services, retail sales, equity prices, and currency demand. Analysis of the effects of the pandemic requires the use of monthly data, as the pandemic was highly concentrated in the single month of October. If the pandemic had notable effects on the economy, then these effects should be apparent in that month, with rebounds occurring in subsequent months.

Monthly data on industrial production are a key source of information on the aggregate impact of the pandemic. To translate this into GNP impacts we regress the annual growth of the Romer real GNP series on annual growth of the NBER index of industrial production and trade. Results are reported in James and Sargent and indicate that a 1 percent change in this index was associated with a 0.26 percent change in GNP.[14]

Figure 17 provides monthly levels of the NBER industrial production index. The pandemic main wave was limited to the September to November period with half the morbidity occurring in October. During the fall wave, industrial production averaged 7 percent below the August level. This translates into a –1.7 percent annual impact and a –0.45 percent GNP impact using the estimated GNP-industrial production elasticity. This may be an overestimate of the pandemic's effect since the First World War ended in November and part of the November weakness likely reflects the cancellation of defence orders. As can be seen in Figure 17, the decline during the fall wave is considerably smaller than declines during normal business-cycle contractions of the period.

FIGURE 17
US: Industrial Production Index, 1913–1922

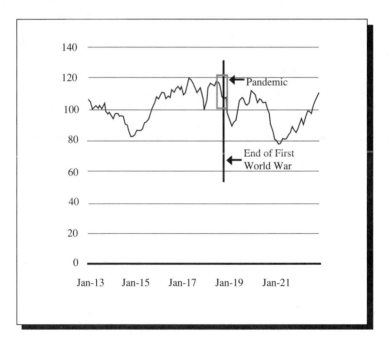

Note: See note to Figure 1.

In the first decades of the twentieth century, the Pullman Company kept detailed data on passenger miles carried, while the City of New York recorded all passenger trips on its subways and street railways. This data, along with monthly retail sales data, allow us to gauge the indirect effects of the pandemic on sectors that could have been vulnerable to psychologically-induced demand reductions. Figures 18 and 19 provide this information relative to the averages of the previous years to control for seasonal effects.

FIGURE 18

Passengers Carried by Pullman Company and New York Transit, 1918–1919

(Jan 1918 = 100, sa)

FIGURE 19

Real US Retail Sales, 1918–1919

(Jan 1918 = 100, sa)

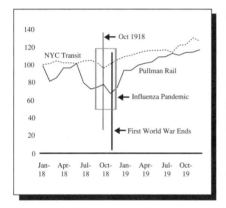

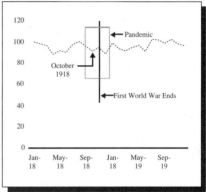

Note: See note to Figure 1.

Pullman rail passenger traffic shows no apparent impact of the pandemic. Traffic was unchanged in September 1918 and actually rose in October, the peak month of the fall wave. A possible pandemic impact is apparent in New York transit use, which rose in September, then fell in October, before recovering in November. The annual impact is small, however, amounting to only –0.6 percent. Retail sales also declined somewhat during the pandemic months, although the decline in October is smaller than the standard deviation of monthly changes in the series. The implied annual impact is –1.4 percent. On balance, the apparent impact of the 1918 pandemic on sensitive sectors ranges between indiscernible and modest.

Some argue that a pandemic would disrupt trade flows. However, as Figure 20 shows, no such impacts were apparent in 1918. While real imports declined modestly during the peak pandemic months, the decline is very small relative to the typical volatility of the series. Real exports were effectively stable.

Kennedy, Thomson and Vujanovic along with the IMF Avian Flu Working Group suggest that a pandemic could negatively affect equity markets and induce people to hoard cash.[15] Again, no such effects were apparent in 1918 (Figures 20 and 21). The Dow-Jones Industrial average was flat during the pandemic while railroad stocks actually increased in value. Rather than leading people to hoard cash, real currency holdings by the public actually fell modestly during the 1918 fall wave. During that year, Americans would have had much greater reason to be nervous about the solvency of their local bank in the event of a negative shock than would be the case today, as bank failures were frequent in the United States prior to the introduction of Federal Deposit Insurance in 1934 and tended to surge during economic downturns.

FIGURE 20   FIGURE 21

US: Real Exports and Imports, 1918–1919   Real US Equity Values and Currency
(deflated by CPI; Jan 1918 = 100)   Holdings, 1918–1919

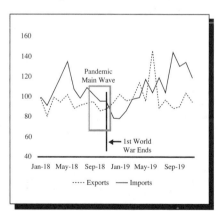
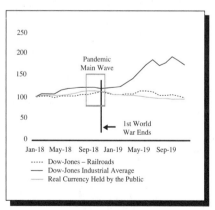

Note: See note to Figure 1.

There is no evidence of any absenteeism-related disruption in the financial sector, as daily bank clearings actually rose (Figure 22). Bankruptcy data show no evidence of any pandemic impact on the financial health of the manufacturing sector (Figure 23).

FIGURE 22

US: Real Daily Bank Clearings, 1918–1919
(monthly average; Jan 1918 = 100)

FIGURE 23

US: Manufacturing Business Failures,
1918–1919

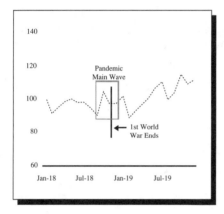

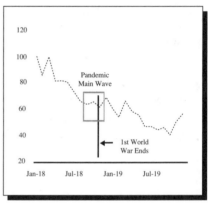

Note: See note to Figure 1.

Overall, the data suggest that the 1918 pandemic had modest direct effects stemming from illness absenteeism, but that indirect effects were very small. This is consistent with the generalized finding of Albala-Bertrand that human activity is very resilient to many natural shocks.[16] People adapt and work around the shock; those unaffected work harder and longer to pick up the slack. The short duration of the shocks also limits their impact. As Alfred Crosby points out:

> Spanish Influenza moved too fast to produce more than brief paralysis. It was a hit-and-run kind of disease, not the kind that places society under a long siege, like tuberculosis or malaria. Influenza does not create the kind of situation which is bound to get worse and worse unless proper actions are taken.[17]

The Economic Impacts of the 1957 and 1968 Pandemics

The 1957 pandemic virus was first identified in East Asia in February 1957. Vaccine production began in May, with limited supplies available in North America by August. Sporadic cases appeared in North America in June; however, the pandemic began in earnest at the beginning of September, with the bulk of morbidity and mortality concentrated in the month of October. A second wave with much lower morbidity began in December even before the first wave had fully run its course. The second wave tailed off in February 1958. As in 1918, most of the impact occurred in one wave, and within that wave, most occurred in a single month.

The North American attack rate in 1957 was around 35 percent with a case mortality rate of 0.12 percent implying population mortality of 0.4 per 1,000. Mortality was concentrated among the very young and very old. Global population mortality is estimated to have been about 0.7 per 1,000.

The 1968 pandemic was milder than that of 1957. The main wave struck in December 1968 with US population mortality at just under 0.2 per 1,000 and global mortality at around 0.3 per 1,000.

The Labour Force Survey of Canada's Dominion Bureau of Statistics recorded monthly illness absenteeism rates throughout the 1950s. Figure 24 provides monthly excess illness absenteeism rates for the years 1955 to 1958. These are calculated as the difference between each month's illness absenteeism rate and the average rate for that month over the years 1955, 1956, 1958, and 1959. The pandemic appears very clearly as a sharp spike in illness absenteeism in the fall of 1957. Excess illness absenteeism rose to 0.7 percent in September, 3.1 percent in the peak month of October, and then fell back to 1.1 percent in November, 0.4 percent in December and January, and 0.2 percent in February. Two distinct waves struck during this period; a main wave lasting from September to November, and a secondary wave from December to February. Calibration of our dynamic morbidity model to the monthly data yields an estimate that daily excess illness absenteeism peaked at 3.8 percent in Canada around 15 October (Figure 25).[18]

Canada and the United States suffered a capital investment recession that began in the late summer of 1957 and ended in the spring of 1958. This recession was preceded by a period of monetary tightening and equity market weakness and was accurately predicted by leading indicators. The recession was characterized by a sharp capital goods inventory cycle.

FIGURE 24

Canadian Actual Excess Illness
Absenteeism, 1955–1958
(percent)

FIGURE 25

Canada: Estimated Daily Excess
Absenteeism Caused by the 1957
Influenza Pandemic (percent)

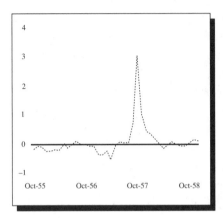

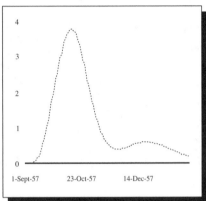

Note: See note to Figure 1.

As in 1918, one must examine monthly data for any signs of economic impact of the pandemic. Figure 26 shows monthly growth of Canadian industrial production and the inverted monthly change in the excess illness absenteeism rate. Industrial production fell 1.9 percent in September 1957, just as the pandemic wave began, with excess absenteeism rising by 0.7 percentage points. Industrial production fell by a smaller 1.1 percent in October and excess absenteeism surged by 2.3 percentage points. In November, industrial production rose by 0.2 percent and excess absenteeism fell by two percentage points.

To try to extract the pandemic signal from the underlying cycle we construct a filtered industrial production series consisting of a five-month centred moving average that excludes October 1957 from the averaging, so as to avoid contamination of the trend with the peak pandemic effect (see Figure 27). Industrial production was 0.7 percent below trend in September 1957, 1.2 percent below in October, and at trend in November. If we take these as the actual pandemic impacts on industrial production, then this implies an annual impact of –0.15 percent. We estimate that the elasticity of real Canadian GDP growth to industrial production growth was 0.58 during the 1950s, yielding an annual GDP impact of –0.08 percent.

FIGURE 26

Canadian Industrial Production and
Excess Illness Absenteeism, 1956–1958

FIGURE 27

Canadian Industrial Production:
Actual and Trend, 1956–1958

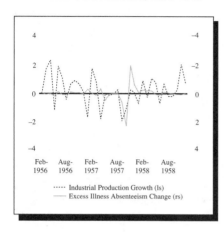

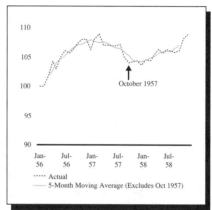

Note: See note to Figure 1. ls = left hand side; rs = right hand side.

No pandemic impacts are apparent in Canadian monthly retail sales (Figure 28). Figure 29 shows the US personal savings rate over the period 1956–69. Any pandemic impacts should appear as a noticeable spike in the pandemic quarter; however, the savings rate actually fell in the fourth quarter of 1957 and was flat in the fourth quarter of 1968. In Canada, even absenteeism rates were unaffected by the 1968 pandemic.

Overall, the picture that emerges from the 1957 and 1968 pandemics is of possible very small direct economic impacts and no indirect impacts.

CONCLUSIONS

We find that the SARS outbreak of 2003 had remarkably little economic impact. Essentially, the effect of SARS was limited to significant but temporary reductions in air travel to affected locations. Hong Kong and Singapore were particularly vulnerable owing to the importance of tourism to their economies. Air travel reductions stemming from SARS and the start of the second Gulf War caused Hong Kong and Singapore GDP to contract in the second quarter of 2003; however, goods trade and retail sales were largely unaffected. Reduced air travel also affected Canada, with negative impacts on the

FIGURE 28

Canada: Real Retail Sales, 1956–1958
(Index; sa)

FIGURE 29

US: Personal Saving Rate, 1956–1969

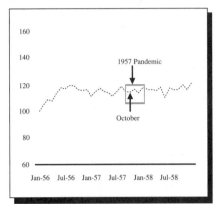

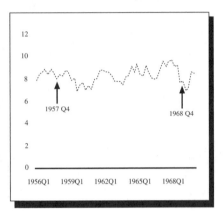

Note: See note to Figure 1.

accommodation industry, particularly in Toronto. Travel and accommodation impacts reduced Canadian annual GDP by only about 0.03 percent in 2003.

A similar conclusion emerges from our analysis of the three major influenza pandemics of the twentieth century. The 1918 influenza pandemic was more severe than any for which we have reliable data. However, US industrial production statistics from the fall of 1918 suggest that the pandemic reduced annual 1918 US GDP by a maximum of 0.5 percent. Only small impacts are apparent in passenger rail and transit use. Retail sales, external trade, financial markets and bankruptcies appear to have been unaffected. The relatively mild 1957 and 1968 pandemics appeared to have very small economic impacts.

Our results are consistent with the broader findings of Albala-Bertrand who examines 28 other natural disasters in 26 countries and finds that the short- and long-run aggregate economic effects are generally much smaller than initially predicted.[19] Effects are small because human societies are extraordinarily adaptable. For almost every direct negative effect there is a potential offsetting response, including economy-wide, sectoral, household, and individual reactions that mitigate the disaster by increasing supplies and changing technologies.

Albala-Bertrand notes that natural disasters usually engender predictions of large negative economic effects, and in particular, large indirect effects. After the fact, effects usually prove small and indirect effects are indiscernible. However, "standing views go largely unchallenged and appear to have a life of their own."[20]

They reflect a view of disasters that "rarely consider the response to disaster impacts as part of the same event — as if society functioned without in-built reactive mechanisms." In fact, "the final outcome of a disaster situation is the net effect of largely negative impact effects and generally positive response effects."[21]

In conclusion, it seems from our analysis of the economic impacts of infectious disease outbreaks in the last one hundred years that human suffering and loss of life far outweigh the effect on the economy. The GDP impacts are not necessarily the best measure of the effects on people of a virus or other natural disaster.

NOTES

The authors wish to thank Alana McDonald, Gloria Wong, Allan Pollock, and Brian Torgunrud for useful input, along with the seminar participants at the UK Health Protection Agency for helpful comments and questions. The views in this paper are those of the authors and should not be attributed to the Department of Finance, Canada.

[1] Sherry Cooper, "The Avian Flu Crisis: An Economic Update," *Bank of Montreal Special Report* (13 March 2006). At www.bmonesbittburns.com/economics/reports/ 20060313/report.pdf; McKibbin and Sidorenko estimate a global GDP impact of –0.8 percent from a mild 1968-type pandemic and –12.6 percent from a pandemic with population mortality roughly double that experienced in 1918; see Warwick J. McKibbin and Alexandra A. Sidorenko, "Global Macroeconomic Consequences of Pandemic Influenza," *Lowry Institute Analysis* (February 2006). At www.brookings .edu/views/papers/mckibbin/ 200602.pdf; The US Congressional Budget Office estimates that a pandemic with population mortality double that of 1918 would reduce the US GDP by 5 percent, while a 1957-type pandemic would reduce GDP by 1.5 percent; see Congressional Budget Office, *A Potential Influenza Pandemic: Possible Macroeconomic Effects and Policy Issues* (December 2005). At www.cbo.gov/ftpdocs/72xx/doc7214/05-22-Avian%20Flu.pdf.

Bloom, de Wit and Carangel-San Jose of the Asian Development Bank estimate that a relatively mild pandemic could reduce Asian GDP by between 2.6 and 6.8 percent, depending on the size of assumed psychological consumption effects; see Erik Bloom, Vincent de Wit and Mary J. Carangel-San Jose, "Potential Economic Impact of an Avian Flu Pandemic on Asia," Asian Development Bank *ERD Policy Brief*, 42 (November 2005). At www.adb.org/Documents/EDRC/Policy_Briefs/PB042.pdf.

Kennedy, Thomson and Vujanovic of the Australian Treasury estimate that a pandemic half as severe as that of 1918 would reduce Australian GDP by 9.3 percent; see Steven Kennedy, Jim Thomson and Petar Vujanovic, "A Primer on the Macroeconomic Effects of an Influenza Pandemic," *Australian Treasury Working Paper 2006-01* (February 2006). At www.treasury.gov.au/documents/1069/PDF/TWP_01_2006.pdf. The New Zealand Treasury estimates that a severe pandemic could reduce GDP by 10 to 20 percent in the year that the pandemic occurred, and by 15 to 30 percent over the medium term; see New Zealand Treasury, *Treasury Report: Avian Influenza Pandemic — Issues* (November 2005). At www.treasury.govt.nz/pandemic/tr05-2024/tr05-2024.pdf.

[2]Bloom, de Wit and Carangel-San Jose, "Potential Economic Impact of an Avian Flu Pandemic on Asia."

[3]World Health Organization (WHO), "Communicable Disease Surveillance and Response, SARS" (Geneva: WHO, 21 April 2004).

[4]Jong-Wha Lee and Warwick J. McKibbin, "Globalisation and Disease: The Case of SARS," Working Paper No. 2003/16 (Canberra: Australian National University, August 2003).

[5]Alan Siu and Richard Y.C. Wong, "Economic Impact of SARS: The Case of Hong Kong," *Asian Economic Papers* 3, no. 1 (Winter 2004):62-83, p. 81.

[6]James Newcomb, "Economic Risks Associated with an Influenza Pandemic." Testimony to the United States Senate Committee on Foreign Relations (November 2005). At http://bio-era.net/Asset/iu_files/Bio-era%20Research%20Reports/Final_testimony_1108_clean.pdf.

[7]For econometric details, see Steven James and Timothy Sargent, "The Economic Impacts of an Influenza Pandemic," Working Paper (Ottawa: Department of Finance, forthcoming 2006).

[8]Emma X. Fan, "SARS: Economic Impacts and Implications," Asian Development Bank *Policy Brief* no. 15 (May 2003), p. 4.

[9]McKibbin and Sidorenko, "Global Macroeconomic Consequences of Pandemic Influenza."

[10]Lee and McKibbin, "Globalisation and Disease," p. 4.

[11]Jin-Tan Liu, James K. Hammitt, Jung-Der Wang and Meng-Wen Tsou, "Valuation of the Risk of SARS in Taiwan." NBER Working Paper No. 10011 (Cambridge, MA: National Bureau of Economic Research, 2003).

[12]J.M. Albala-Bertrand, *Political Economy of Large Natural Disasters: With Special Reference to Developing Countries* (New York: Oxford University Press, 1993).

[13]See, for example, Joel Slemrod, "Thanatology and Economics: The Behavioral Economics of Death," *AEA Papers and Proceedings* 93, no. 2 (May 2003):371-75.

[14]James and Sargent, "The Economic Impacts of an Influenza Pandemic," Table D.4 of Annex D.

[15]Kennedy, Thomson and Vujanovic, "A Primer on the Macroeconomic Effects of an Influenza Pandemic." IMF Avian Flu Working Group, "The Global Economic and Financial Impact of an Avian Flu Pandemic and the Role of the IMF," (2006). At www.imf.org/external/pubs/ft/afp/2006/eng/022806.pdf.

[16]Albala-Bertrand, *Political Economy of Large Natural Disasters.*

[17]Alfred W. Crosby, *America's Forgotten Pandemic: The Influenza of 1918*, 2nd edition (Cambridge: Cambridge University Press, 2003), p. 115.

[18]See James and Sargent, "The Economic Impacts of an Influenza Pandemic," for details.

[19]Albala-Bertrand, *Political Economy of Large Natural Disasters.*

[20]Ibid., p. 3.

[21]Ibid., p. 10.

About the Authors

ANN G. CARMICHAEL, MD PhD, is Associate Professor at Indiana University, Bloomington. She is the author of *Plague and the Poor in Renaissance Florence* (Cambridge and New York: Cambridge University Press, 1986) and editor with Richard M. Ratzan of *Medicine: A Treasury of Art and Literature* (New York: Hugh Lauter Levin Associates, Distributed by Macmillan, 1991).

K. CODELL CARTER, PhD, is Professor of Philosophy at Brigham Young University, Provo. He is the author of *The Rise of Causal Concepts of Disease: Case Histories* (Aldershot and Burlington, VT: Ashgate, 2003); and with Barbara R. Carter, *Childbed Fever: A Scientific Biography of Ignaz Semmelweis* (Westport, CT: Greenwood Press, 1994). He has also translated and edited, *Essays of Robert Koch* (New York: Greenwood Press, 1987) and *The Etiology, Concept, and Prophylaxis of Childbed Fever* by Ignaz Semmelweis (Madison, WI: University of Wisconsin Press, 1983).

JAY CASSEL, PhD, studied at Oxford and the University of Toronto. He has taught history at several universities, and has worked on television documentaries for CBC, PBS, and National Geographic. He is the author of *The Secret Plague: Venereal Disease in Canada, 1838–1939* (Toronto: University of Toronto Press, 1987).

JACALYN DUFFIN, MD PhD, is the Hannah Professor of the History of Medicine at Queen's University, Kingston. She is the author of *Langstaff: A Nineteenth-Century Medical Life* (Toronto: University of Toronto Press, 1993), *To See with a Better Eye: A Life of RTH Laennec* (Princeton, NJ: Princeton University Press, 1998), *History of Medicine: A Scandalously Short Introduction*

(Toronto: University of Toronto Press 1999), *Lovers and Livers: Disease Concepts in History* (Toronto: University of Toronto Press, 2005), and (as editor) *Clio in the Clinic: Doctors Stories of History in Medical Practice* (Oxford and Toronto: Oxford University Press and University of Toronto Press, 2005).

GEORGINA FELDBERG, PhD, is Associate Professor of Social Science at York University, Toronto. She is the author of *Disease and Class: Tuberculosis and the Shaping of Modern North American Society* (New Brunswick: Rutgers University Press, 1995) and a co-editor of *Women, Health and Nation: Canada and the United States since 1945* (Montreal and Kingston: McGill-Queen's University Press/Associated Medical Services [Hannah Institute], 2003).

STEVEN JAMES obtained both a BA and an MA in Economics from the University of British Columbia and pursued doctoral studies at Princeton University. He joined the Department of Finance in 1987, and is now Director of the Economic Analysis and Forecasting Division, which is responsible for analyzing economic developments in the Canadian, US, and overseas economies.

HARVEY LAZAR, PhD, is senior research associate at the Centre for Global Studies at the University of Victoria. A graduate of the London School of Economics and Political Science, he had a long career in the Canadian public service, including the Economic Council of Canada and Human Resources Development Canada. He served as Director of the Institute of Intergovernmental Relations at Queen's University from 1997 to 2005. During his years in public service, he contributed to research reports on such diverse topics as retirement income policy, social policy, and labour market development. His current work focuses on Canadian and comparative federalism, including the Canadian social union, health governance, and fiscal federalism.

HEATHER A. MACDOUGALL, PhD, is Associate Professor of History at the University of Waterloo, where, from 2000 to 2005, she also served as Associate Dean of Arts for Graduate Studies and Research. She is the author of *Activists and Advocates: Toronto's Health Department, 1883–1983* (Toronto: Dundurn Press, 1990). Her current work focuses on the history of the Canadian medicare program and on evolving policy in public health and disease control.

TIMOTHY SARGENT is an economist with a BA from the University of Manchester, an MA from the University of Western Ontario, and a PhD (1995) from the University of British Columbia. He joined the Department of Finance in 1994, where he is Senior Chief in the Economic Analysis and Forecasting Division, which is responsible for analyzing economic developments in the Canadian, US, and overseas economies.

ARTHUR SWEETMAN, PhD, is an economist and Director of the School of Policy Studies at Queen's University, Kingston where he holds the Stauffer-Dunning Chair. His research interests are in economic issues related to labour markets, education, and health policy.

KUMANAN WILSON, MD, MSc, is a specialist in general internal medicine at the Toronto General Hospital and associate professor in the Departments of Medicine and Health Policy, Management and Evaluation at the University of Toronto. He is also a Research Associate at the Institute of Intergovernmental Relations at Queen's University and a member of the Joint Centre for Bioethics, University of Toronto. A medical graduate of the University of Western Ontario, he did his residency and graduate work in health research methods at McMaster University. As a Canadian Institutes of Health Research (CIHR) New Investigator, Dr. Wilson focuses on policy-making in areas of health protection, such as Canadian immunization policy, decision-making in the Canadian blood system, and the impact of intergovernmental relations on health policy. He is currently examining the impact of federalism on public health.

JAMES G. YOUNG, MD, was appointed Chief Coroner and General Inspector of Anatomy for the province of Ontario in 1990. In 1994, he was named Assistant Deputy Minister, Public Safety Division, Ministry of Public Safety and Security and on 26 June 2002, he was appointed Ontario's first Commissioner of Public Security, a title changed on 26 June 2003, to Commissioner of Public Safety and Security. During the SARS outbreaks in the spring of 2003, Dr. Young was the co-manager of the provincial emergency and was responsible for providing leadership and coordinating activities to manage and control the outbreaks. He also served as one of the government's spokespersons in daily briefings with the press.

DICK ZOUTMAN, MD, is Professor in the Departments of Pathology and Molecular Medicine, of Community Health and Epidemiology, and of Medicine at Queen's University, Kingston. He serves as Chief of Medical Microbiology and Infection Control of Kingston General Hospital, and chairs the Division of Infectious Disease within the Department of Medicine.

INDEX